Dancing Fear & Desire

Race, Sexuality, and Imperial Politics
in Middle Eastern Dance

Cultural Studies Series

Cultural Studies is the multi- and interdisciplinary study of culture, defined anthropologically as a "way of life," performatively as symbolic practice, and ideologically as the collective product of media and cultural industries, i.e., pop culture. Although Cultural Studies is a relative newcomer to the humanities and social sciences, in less than half a century it has taken interdisciplinary scholarship to a new level of sophistication, reinvigorating the liberal arts curriculum with new theories, new topics, and new forms of intellectual partnership.

The Cultural Studies series includes topics such as construction of identities; regionalism/nationalism cultural citizenship; migration; popular culture; consumer cultures; media and film; the body; postcolonial criticism; cultural policy; sexualities; cultural theory; youth culture; class relations; and gender.

The new Cultural Studies series from Wilfrid Laurier University Press invites submission of manuscripts concerned with critical discussions on power relations concerning gender, class, sexual preference, ethnicity, and other macro and micro sites of political struggle.

For further information, please contact the Series Editor:
Jodey Castricano
Department of English
Wilfrid Laurier University Press
75 University Avenue West
Waterloo, Ontario, Canada, N2L 3C5

Dancing Fear & Desire

Race, Sexuality, and Imperial Politics
in Middle Eastern Dance

Stavros Stavrou Karayanni

Wilfrid Laurier University Press

We acknowledge the financial support of the Government of Canada through the Book Publishing Industry Development Program for our publishing activities. We acknowledge the Government of Ontario through the Ontario Media Development Corporation's Ontario Book Initiative.

Library and Archives Canada Cataloguing in Publication

Karayanni, Stavros Stavrou, 1965–
    Dancing fear and desire : race, sexuality, and imperial politics in Middle Eastern dance / Stavros Stavrou Karayanni.

(Cultural studies series)
Includes bibliographical references and index.
ISBN 0-88920-454-3

1. Belly dance—Middle East. 2. Belly dance—Greece. 3. Belly dance—Political aspects. 4. Belly dance—Social aspects. 5. Gender identity in dance. 6. Homosexuality and dance. 7. Male dancers. I. Title. II. Series: Cultural studies series (Waterloo, Ont.)

GV1798.5.K37 2004   793.3   C2004-905761-8

Cover and text design by P.J. Woodland. Cover photograph of Cihangir Gümüstürkmen by Daniela Incoronato.

Printed in Canada

Order from:
Wilfrid Laurier University Press
Wilfrid Laurier University
Waterloo, Ontario, Canada N2L 3C5
www.wlupress.wlu.ca

αφιερωμένη αυτή η προσπάθεια στην μνήμη της γιαγιάς μου Ουρανίας, που με έμαθε γράμματα και την αξία της εξιστόρησης,

και στην Μαρίζα Κώχ που μου χάρισε έκφραση και με δίδαξε την συγκίνηση και την αγάπη για τήν τέχνη

Table of Contents

Acknowledgements

I have been extremely fortunate and blessed to have a very special family of friends who have offered me support, collaboration, and assistance. This project would not have materialized without them. I thank Smaro Kamboureli who in March 1998 promised me that such a topic would be interesting and urged me to undertake this research. I am indebted to her encouragement, advice, and support throughout this project. I am also grateful to Aruna Srivastava, whose guidance and generosity kept me going; and to Ashok Mathur for good humour and advice. Thanks also to David Bateman, Susan Bennett, Anne Flynn, Brent Craig, Khang Nguyen, Sharron Proulx, Hiromi Goto, and Cristina Glaeser.

I am also indebted to people whom I proudly call my "international dance family" whose members range from people I know well and have been friends with to people I have only met virtually until now. All of them, however, have been wonderfully supportive of this project as well as of my presence in the belly dance community. Shareen el-Safy and Ron Iverson have promoted my work in *Habibi*. Artemis Mourat provided images; Kristina Robyn in Sydney, Australia, offered dancing, hospitality, and warm friendship; Elena Marie Villa provided material support; Yasmina Ramzy and Jalilah have been wonderful and giving dance instructors, dance lovers, and dance scholars; and Julian Awwad shared electric shimmies and stimulating discussions on belly dance.

I am grateful to Alkis Raftis, president of the Conseil International de la Danse (CID), for supporting my work. He works with an Athenian troupe of wonderful people who have been generous towards me, especially Anastasia Romveli. I am particularly indebted to Anthony Shay for his numerous and valuable contributions to *Dance Studies* and for indispensable advice, support, and feedback. And I thank Cihangir Gümüsturkmen for sharing his fabulous work, especially the photo on the cover of this book.

*Acknow-
ledgements*

Jacqueline Larson at Wilfrid Laurier Press guided me through the various critical stages of this book. She has believed in this work with a confidence that breathed fresh life into it. Finally, I thank my family, and especially Anthi Sideropoulou, for not refusing any help I requested, and my mother Anthoulla for her gorgeous singing, artistic sensibility, and selfless sacrifices and struggles that she continues to endure—without complaint—for all her children.

I dedicate this work to two women of great accomplishment and also great influence in my life: my grandmother Ourania who taught me how to read and listen to stories. And to Mariza Koch who through her artistry taught me to love and appreciate art. In her voice I was born into a new awareness of my body and sensibility.

Grateful acknowledgements for permission to reprint from *The Letters of Gustave Flaubert: Volume 1, 1830-1857*, selected, edited, and translated by Francis Steegmuller, 110-11 (Cambridge, MA: Belknap Press of Harvard University Press, Copyright ©1979, 1980 by Francis Steegmuller). Also from *Manners and Customs of the Modern Egyptians* by Edward W. Lane (1908) by permission of Everyman's Library.

Part of chapter 2 was originally published, in a substantially altered form, in *Habibi* 19.1 (January 2002): 18-21. Also, an early and short version of chapter 5 appeared in *Dance as Intangible Heritage*, edited by Alkis Raftis (Athens: Tropos Zois, 2002), 75-84. Finally, I included brief excerpts from chapter 1 and the epilogue in the article "Cyprus after History" co-authored with Spurgeon Thompson and Myria Vassiliadou for *Interventions: International Journal of Postcolonial Studies* 6.2 (June 2004): 282-99.

Preface

The genesis of this project has had a long incubation that spans several years of emotional and intellectual involvement with issues of belonging, nationality, and the performance of gender and sexuality. Spiralling through these political issues and performances was the body of belly dance, intransigent and seductive, moving in all the formidability of the contradictory reconstructions that it has undergone in its twentieth-century troubled history—derided and adored, abandoned and retrieved, abused and exalted. I have known it and loved it and wanted it for as long as I can remember, yet for various reasons related to the prejudices attached to a man belly dancing but also connected to issues of ethnic and racial identity, I made it to a dance workshop in Calgary only at the age of thirty-three. So this is a book about unfulfilled passions and yearning, but also about belated epiphanies that weave themselves into a textual choreography.

I wanted to produce work that could accommodate my specific concerns with various forms of oppression and with the appropriation of expression while addressing and exploring mediums of resistance. Western academic discourse has, fortunately, permitted the creation of a space that can accommodate the voice of a queer person from an ex-colony— a person whose colonization continues in myriad ways at home and who has come to a profound investment in movement as a marker of identity and expression. Sadly, my own country's postcolonial social and cultural politics exclude me completely from their concerns and exile me, deliberately and methodically, into disenfranchised spaces where, if citizenship denotes a privilege of belonging, then this privilege remains an undelivered gift. Hence the dual and parallel trajectory that the book follows: it experiments with critical autobiography but it also relies on the deployment of critical theory in its investigation. In the pages that follow, there-

     Notes to preface are on page 199.

fore, I bring to the forefront—and at times privilege—texts that are wildly heterogeneous: memories of events and persons, historical circumstances, travel narratives, letters and correspondence, film and video, newspaper articles, as well as a close look at Oscar Wilde's play *Salomé*. In my reading of these texts, I rely heavily on the use of theoretical tools that I borrow from critics whose work has advanced the discourse of postcolonial, dance, and queer theory. In bringing together such a range of texts, I hope to demonstrate how dance moves across that complex and uneven stage where diverse textual, social, and cultural practices perform their histrionics. The organization of social life, or cultural hegemony, is rehearsed, maintained, challenged, and ultimately transformed on this stage while movement registers, affects, and inflects every detail of this transformation. My argument is bifurcated: I examine the often elaborate procedures through which Middle Eastern dance (popularly known as belly dance) has been the object of cultural appropriation, manipulated into complicity by an Orientalist agenda. At the same time, however, this same art form incorporates a rare and unyielding potential (or promise) for various kinds of resistances: social, cultural, sexual.

In its initial conception, I intended this project to investigate and interrogate various travel narratives where Middle Eastern dancers appeared and danced only to vanish behind a curtain of ideological conceits and (mostly male) censuring remarks. Now I realize that such a project, although promising, would have to struggle against tedium since many of the narratives repeat the same images so that the dance is buried beneath a growing mound of tautological signifiers. What rescued me from this potential trauma was "the Greek stuff" that invited itself into my project, pleading yet unyielding, imperceptible yet emphatic. An examination of Oriental dancers and their encounters with Western colonial (and often sexual) hunger would probably produce a neat critical argument. However, the (almost imperative) inclusion of my own politics of nation and sexual identity have untidied the project since they required my own location in discursive history. They have also mobilized different forces, not merely for the purpose of understanding political oppression but for designating sites of resistance as well.

Perhaps it is not surprising then that one of the challenges has been to make this project cohere for the reader. One may find, for example, that there seems to be no apparent connection between European narratives about Middle Eastern dancers and Greek politics of identity. Although I feel that I embody these connections, the challenge has been to articu-

late them in a consistent theoretical framework and produce a service-
able argument. In writing about the unruly interimplications of dance
movement and identity embodiment, one quickly discovers that neat,
symmetrical formulas are not easy to apply, nor are they desirable. If there
is a main unifying approach then, it can be traced to a textual reading of
choreographic movement, a treatment, in other words, of (dance) movement as text. I am concerned with the politics of dance—tsifteteli, belly
dance, Oriental dance (I provide a detailed discussion of these terms in
the section entitled "Some Notes on the Terms" in chapter 1)—and those
controversial moves common to all these variations, moves that signify
transgression by giving voice to parts of the body that are expected to
remain silent, unobtrusive, and discomfited in their postcolonial posture.
I look at dancing bodies that arouse emotion in the viewer and I examine how their movements are defined by and in turn define imperial interests as these negotiate the construction of masculine and feminine
subjectivities, sexualities, and nationhood. Predictably, then, this project
pulls me into all directions, leading me into a lengthy and unforeseen
improvisation whose theme emerged only piecemeal through the length
of its possessing and possessed choreography.

A passage from Susan Foster's landmark essay "Choreographing History," assists and refines my purpose.

> At some point, historical bodies that have formed in the imagination and
> on the written page seem to take on a life of their own. The historical
> inquiry takes on sufficient structure and energy to generate meaning and
> to narrate itself. Its representational and narrational determinants, infused
> with their author's energy and with the vibrancy of dead bodies, begin to
> perambulate on their own. (10)

I am hoping to give voice to silent moments and imbue gestures with
energy so that they begin to narrate themselves; or, in Foster's terms, the
representational and narrational determinants of my personal and historical inquiry will gather momentum and perform their significance with a
will of their own. What Foster suggests and what I strive for in this book
does suggest processes that are, indeed, dependent on a magical quality
embedded in the transformations afforded by the body of dance as it
inter-implicates with the dance of the body.

"Who cares about the tsifteteli?" a Greek friend protested after reading a very early draft of the work, with a tone of exasperation that, in
effect, spelled out censorious admonition to my endeavour. And, integrat-
ing a personal dimension to her critique, she proceeded to exclaim: "And

stop talking about yourself all the time—it's annoying. This is academic work and not a critical memoir. How are you advancing the discourse?" (She pronounced it "diskôrs.")[1] Such response frightens and immobilizes me completely. It pushes me back into the confinement of my colonized body—colonized by a British administration whose legacy has been emulated by the Cyprus Republic and the extremely powerful Orthodox Church of Cyprus, whose work on policing performances of ethnicity, gender, class, and sexuality have been totalizing in their success. After dismissing the tsifteteli—a dance that can be a vital form of artistic expression—as unworthy of scholarly attention and annihilating its potential for alternative, liberating performances, my friend proceeded to isolate me further in an abstract "academic" space where my body, in effect my historiography, was immaterial before the mandate of a larger, more significant but nondescript academic project on some other traditionally acceptable, and therefore legitimate topic. I find it necessary to refer to her objections here because they are, unfortunately, a concise summation of the various oppressions that have shaped my identity. Such objections derive from identification with a supremacy that is made nervous by bodies like mine, which are, as a result, silenced and bullied into withdrawal.

This work, therefore, emerges from personal interpellation and in some ways its writing exorcises the violent image repertoire that haunted my childhood in Cyprus; more specifically, the post-independence flaring of hatred and fighting between the Turkish and Greek communities of the island, the coup d'état and subsequent invasion of Turkish troops in 1974, as well as my own sexual oppression. I was born months after my father was murdered during the intercommunal clashes of 1963, so my birth was also my introduction into an environment of loss and mourning.[2] His dead body shadowed my childhood with its enormous absence, like some painful, distended mystery that taunted me with meanings that were supposed to be patently transparent, yet confounded me with their inexplicability. It was clear who the enemy was and how I was expected to respond—hence the transparency—yet this "clarity" never ceased to engender questioning in my mind. The politics constructed around this portentous event wanted me positioned against the "Turk" and determined an embodiment that I have not lived up to in several ways. Instead, I have needed to retrace some of the connections I share with Arabs and Turks, my geographical neighbours and cultural relatives, connections that were severed in the contemporary postcolonial context. In a sense, my desire to carry out historical research on dancers in the Middle East seeks to satisfy the need to reclaim some of what I feel I have always been entitled to. Therefore, the dance tradition of the Greek tsifteteli becomes for a Cypriot like me a crossroads of sorts: a meeting point that reconciles politics of gender, sexuality, nation, and race. Yet, this dance is never a fixed crossroads point. It has the capacity to flow into all the spaces opened up by grief and loss, joy and exaltation, and moves them in a concerted kinesthesia.

1 / Introducing Colonial
and Postcolonial Dialectics
on the Subject of Dance

Oh my body, make of me always a man who questions!
Frantz Fanon, Black Skin, White Masks

The space I occupy might be explained by my history. It is a position into which I have been written. I am not privileging it, but I do want to use it. I can't fully construct a position that is different from the one I am in.
Gayatri Spivak, The Postcolonial Critic

So ubiquitous, so "naturalized" as to be nearly unnoticed as a symbolic system, movement is a primary not secondary social "text"—complex, polysemous, already always meaningful, yet continuously changing. Its articulation signals group affiliation and group differences, whether consciously performed or not. Movement serves as a marker for the production of gender, racial, ethnic, class, and national identities. It can also be read as a signal of sexual identity, age, and illness or health, as well as various other types of distinctions/descriptions that are applied to individuals or groups, such as "sexy."
Jane C. Desmond, "Embodying Difference:
Issues in Dance and Cultural Studies"

   Notes to chapter 1 are on page 199.

2

Introducing
Colonial and
Postcolonial
Dialectics
on the
Subject
of Dance

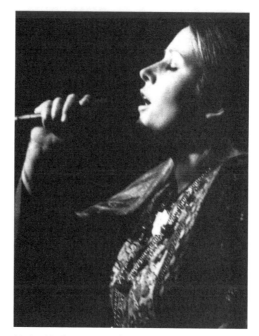

Mariza Koch. 1976. (author's private collection)

The year is 1976 and The Hague in Holland is hosting the Eurovision Song Contest. The 1974 events in Cyprus, the coup d'état
by the Greek junta supported and aided by Greek-Cypriot right-
wing nationalists, and the subsequent invasion of the island by Turkish
troops, are still a fresh and open wound for Greeks. An island where the
communities once cohabited in mixed villages is now divided into a Greek
South and a Turkish North, an extremely painful division that, apart
from being politically unacceptable, also marks the breakdown of possibilities for reconciliation between the two communities. Greece, with
Manos Hadjidakis as the State TV and Radio Director, takes the adroit
decision to participate in the Eurovision Song Contest with a distinctly
politicized entry, a song that mourns the destruction of the island and
decries the injustice against the people of Cyprus.[1] Mariza Koch, the singer who performs the controversial song, receives several threats before
as well as on the evening of the contest, which are presumably intended
to frighten her into withdrawing even at the last minute.[2] She persists
and appears on stage in a long black dress in a solemn and composed
attitude. Next to her, a lagouto player accompanies her singing.[3]

Introducting
Colonial and
Postcolonial
Dialectics
on the
Subject
of Dance

I invoke this performative moment because its powerful significations demand that it be resituated and reassessed in postcolonial cultural history. As with many important moments in Greek culture, the full implications of this event remain unexamined.[4] In terms of my interest here, the 1976 Eurovision Song Festival becomes the confluence of several narratives that have come to affect, directly and indirectly, my involvement with Middle Eastern dance. With the song being quite clearly an outcry against Turkish foreign policy, Turkish state television interrupts the live transmission and replaces the Greek entry with a belly dance performance—at least this was the report in some Cypriot newspapers. Shortly after the contest, the Greek Cypriot newspaper *Fileleftheros* published a poem by Diogenis, a popular satirical poet, in which the reader was expected to find humour in the contrast between Koch's appearance and belly dancing, which the poem depicted in terms of excess and grotesqueness: "to be liked by the Turks Mariza should have tossed her belly to *other* rhythms/… shaking her bottom just like Emine" [a female name easily recognized as Turkish by Greek Cypriots] (1, my emphasis, my translation).

On the level of nationalism, this moment foregrounded "Greekness" in all its complex and irresolute meanings. The presentation of the Greek entry in 1976 provided grounds for protest from those Greek sections that had surrendered to this ideology of "cosmopolitanism." In Greece and Cyprus, public opinion on the song's character and scope was deeply divided. Many critiqued the artist and her colleagues for participating in a "cosmopolitan" international musical contest with a song whose strongly political content, they believed, rendered it inappropriate for Eurovision standards and certainly inadequate to express the "mood" and "atmosphere" of the event. In a gesture that clearly defied such imperatives, Mariza Koch performed an embodiment that was subtle yet provocative. To those Greeks who protested the entry, the song's presentation seemed an audacious intervention in the glitzy Eurovision spectacle. In her black dress and solemn posture, both appropriate for the lamenting lyrics, Mariza Koch embodied a certain folkloric musical tradition through gestures that formed an unapologetic and unromantic composition.[5] While by this point tourism popularized the bouzouki (a popular Greek instrument) as a ubiquitous signifier of Greek fun and entertainment, the lagouto existed in a more remote folkloric context.[6] Moreover, its presence on the Eurovision stage was not decorative and neither was the instrument treated as a relic that vaguely referred to the "exotic." Instead, it had a definitive function that did not rely—as the bouzouki would in such a case—on the

4

*Introducing
Colonial and
Postcolonial
Dialectics
on the
Subject
of Dance*

evocation of a familiar sound associated with Greek tavernas and a certain touristic nostalgia that such an evocation might induce abroad. Furthermore, although born in Athens, Mariza Koch grew up on the island of Santorini in the 1950s, when the voice of instruments such as the lagouto expressed social and cultural history and acted as an integral agent in the historic narrative of the community's past and present. Therefore, although referencing tradition abroad might often be an undeniably romantic gesture, the signifiers that were mobilized denied the audience easy assimilation of the experience.[7]

This introduction to the colonial and postcolonial dialectics on dance is rather ambitious in its scope. It hopes to accomplish a number of tasks that I will divide into five sections. The first section, "Dancing Identity Politics," examines the theoretical implications of the specific Eurovision event that I open with and then expands on the national meanings generated by Koch's performance. My exegesis of the event relies on personal narrative and reflection on the issues, a methodological approach that determines my investigation into the overarching questions about national identity, sexuality, and dance performance. The next section, "Colonial Definitions of Acceptable Performance," examines events in culture and in history, trying to locate the parameters of sexual, national, and racial performance in Cyprus, an excolonized island. In my examination, I seize various opportunities to narrate and explore personal records and memories. Rather appropriately, then, the third section, "Performing Theory," addresses the issue of my casting theoretical considerations in an autobiographical light. Because this project explores a territory where disciplines, methodologies, and concerns are varied, dealing with the nomenclature has been a major challenge. Providing a glossary did not seem a good option since the terms I use cannot be adequately explicated in straightforward definitions. More often than not, they are laden with political implications, complications, and deliberate equivocations, so instead of a glossary I have opted for a discursive analysis that will at least broach the issues and politics of the terms that are fundamental in this work. This attempt forms the fourth section of this chapter and is entitled, "Some Notes on the Terms." The final section, as its subtitle denotes, offers a preview of chapter-by-chapter organization that underlies the book's focus on the sexual, racial, and imperial politics of identity performance.

Dancing Identity Politics

The Eurovision Song Contest's appeal was—and continues to be—founded on a certain cosmopolitan flair. "Cosmopolitan" is a term with significations that have endowed it with an unusual legitimacy in post-colonial Europe. While the Eurovision is an event that presumably celebrates the musical production of various states, its stage has been an exposition ground for international politics as well as a reassertion of metropolitan privilege. Western European countries, particularly England, France, and Germany, have been among the most frequent winners, a status that has permitted them the pose of cultural champions that set pan-European standards (a pose that has looked rather awkward on Ireland which also won the contest several times). Especially in the 1970s and the '80s, these pan-European standards were the cover for encouraging tedious artistic output, superficial and inconsequential musical compositions that, under the guise of "successful" pop songs, were (and continue to be) in accord with the interests of a global order of things where indigenous character is immaterial.[8] In my estimation, the Eurovision Song Contest is yet another imperial endeavour with a neo-colonialist function in modern Europe. It camouflages as an event that celebrates the musical diversity of Europe, but reasserts, in effect, the dominance of its Western members under the guise of "cosmopolitanism."

Mariza Koch with her song's politics configured domestic and international cultural issues by thematizing the 1974 war in Cyprus and condemning the continuing occupation by Turkish troops of the northern part of the island. With sadness, I watched on television and read in the newspapers how a part of the Greek and Cypriot public deemed the song and its presentation inappropriate. The debate over the character of Greek musical tradition had been raging for awhile and Greece felt compelled, pressured even, to somehow match Western Europe in artistic level and cultural production.[9] In fact, the competition engendered a certain vague embarrassment about Greek folk tradition, whose very existence was often regarded as an impediment in the struggle to achieve the progress signified by Western Europe and its arts. Therefore, Mariza Koch's participation in the contest with a traditional song rendered with a folk musical instrument provoked the complexes that marked the relationship of many Greeks with their native culture.

In 1976, I was eleven years old, with the memory of the war still vivid and with painful questions pushing hard against the walls of my mind. Yet I was also quite preoccupied with personal passions that

Introducing
Colonial and
Postcolonial
Dialectics
on the
Subject
of Dance

impinged on these larger concerns. I was obsessively and hopelessly enamoured with Mariza Koch. Some inexplicable power, whose swaying force was religious in its devotion and intensity, was urging me to worship this female singer with that keen and rare devotion that sprung from a desperate need to seek expression for my difference. In an upbringing weighed down by the exigencies of the ethnic conflict, the terror of the war, and my own personal struggles with the oppressions of a postcolonial, heterosexist, and patriarchal regime, Mariza became not the answer to my painful questions but the artistic vision that offered me corporeal awareness and an artistic sensibility. Her voice and her embodiment of art carried an expressive relation to my body. In Wayne Koestenbaum's terms, "the dance of sound waves on the tympanum" (42), and my sympathetic identification with the singer assisted me in reclaiming for myself the body that straight socialization made me discard.[10] Therefore, I felt content to be compelled by the contagion of her presence and operatic voice, unique among Greek singers.[11] My imagination became completely inundated with an image and a voice that came to mitigate, alleviate even, the censorship I felt subjected to by articulating a desire for expression and by granting me permission to love this artist excessively, or to put it differently, "queerly."[12]

At the time, the messages of the Eurovision Song Contest, although complex, were clear even to an eleven-year-old. Even though Mariza's entry was a plea for the suffering of Cypriots and the disaster of the war, there were objections from the very people whom the song supported. I had to contend with the view that traditional instruments and operatic singers who perform folk-inspired songs in a European song contest could not usher in cultural progress. Second, Turkey, which, in the discourse of Greek-Cypriot nationalism, was believed to be a barbaric and backward nation, insulted the Greeks once again by refusing to broadcast our entry.[13] In the Greek nationalist imaginary, more than surprise or outrage, this insult came to reinforce existing racist notions of Turkish culture.

One might expect that a book focusing on dance and politics would be more likely to open with a description of a dance performance rather than singing. I would argue, however, that there are ways to observe singing as a performance of the body, not necessarily because the singer dances but because singing is also an embodied art form with the body carrying not movement but a voice that resonates in the physical realm, transforming it as movement in physical space. Moreover, my account seeks to allow the event to perform itself as I choreograph it in my context. Through this performance, I manoeuvre, indirectly, the introduction of my own body in the work, since my corporeal awareness is directly linked to Mariza Koch as inspiration, escape, and artistic embodiment. In fact, I perceive my performance of and direction of my narrative as signs of my queerness in the way that Eve Kosofsky Sedgwick describes:

> I think that for many of us in childhood the ability to attach intently to a few cultural objects, objects of high or popular culture or both, objects whose meaning seemed mysterious, excessive, or oblique in relation to the codes most readily available to us, became a prime resource for survival. We needed for there to be sites where meanings didn't line up tidily with each other, and we learned to invest those sites with fascination and love. (*Tendencies* 3)

My love for Mariza Koch (an exponent of high as well as popular culture) provided the means to create a site where my very own, and still inchoate, meanings could be accommodated. This love was "mysterious, excessive," asserting itself in an environment where emotional investment in such meanings was neither encouraged nor respected—especially for boys.

Similarly, Sedgwick's remark on the untidy lining up of these meanings materializes in my secret fascination with belly dance. The dancer in the belly dance show that replaced the Greek entry on Turkish television figured in my mind as a confused signifier, alluring and appalling at once. Nevertheless, even though I had never seen this particular show, I felt pressured by the expectation to denounce and deplore such cultural demonstrations. If I introduce the dance itself in this project in a manner that is muted and rather unceremonial—the "other" performance to Mariza Koch's—then this is a reflection of its awkward, uncomfortable, and ultimately silenced form in which I received it. The devotion I nurtured for Mariza became a means to acquire awareness and expression for my body, while belly dance complemented my resistance to normalization by becoming a passionate worship with its own distinct acts of ritual. I revelled in its possibilities as I secretly gyrated my hips, and indulged my imagination in a voluptuous vision of my body. This was a taboo dance for a boy, and my childhood fascination with it was nothing less than aberrance. Yet it was also empowering in a sense, so I kept turning the dial on the radio at home to listen to Arabic radio stations, an indulgence in the foreign and exotic culture that was quite close geographically and yet far away, forcefully distanced by political ideologies. While I envisioned the moves, my ears drank in the melodies and the

*Introducing
Colonial and
Postcolonial
Dialectics
on the
Subject
of Dance*

maqams, or musical roads, which were as familiar to my sensibility as the family features that you recognize in a close relative with whom you are not on speaking terms because of family feuds. Loving that which was proscribed, and in a manner that was censored, became a means of resisting my construction by assuming another "devious" identity. What I knew about belly dance was very little but enough at the same time to make it appear absolutely enchanting in my eyes, although its tradition, as well as its expressive possibilities, remained obscure because of the cultural dictatorship under which I was seeking inspiration for my creativity.

This cultural dictatorship was the implementation of an unrelenting Greek Cypriot nationalism that sought to assuage its anxieties about identity by normalizing all things Cypriot according to the vague and undefined dogma of Greekness. Of course, Greece's own place in the East/West divide has been equivocal, even though in the language of international diplomacy Greece has firmly identified as "European." Greek territorial and economic struggles signified a certain vulnerability and evoked the sensitive and ever-haunting issue of national identity and belonging. Western constructions of Greece often situated it in an indeterminate or ambivalent space in the East/West dichotomy. Greece's relationship with the metropolis is succinctly articulated by Mr. Beebe in E.M. Forster's *A Room with a View*: "Italy is heroic, but Greece is godlike or devilish—I am not sure which, and in either case absolutely out of our suburban focus.... If our poor little Cockney lives must have a background, let it be Italian" (197). Michael Herzfeld locates this ambivalence also in the Greek attitude to "Europe." On the one hand, Europe is a geographical and cultural site where Greeks belong, while, on the other, "Europe" is a concept that remains foreign, distant, and incomprehensible: "such oscillation between two models is not the result of some 'constant inconstancy of the Greek character' but a linguistic and conceptual adaptation to the conflict between an imported ideology and a nativist one" (*Ours Once More* 21).[14]

Perhaps it was this equivocation that enabled Greek sensibility to accept certain traditions while simultaneously isolating these same traditions into something that is strongly reminiscent of Anne McClintock's trope of "anachronistic space." This invention, McClintock argues, "reached full authority as an administrative and regulatory technology in the late Victorian era. Within this trope, the agency of women, the colonized and the industrial working class are disavowed and projected onto anachronistic space: prehistoric, atavistic and irrational, inherently out of place in the historical time of modernity" (40).

The lessons of imperial "progress" instructed Greek sensibility to regard Mariza Koch's participation in the Eurovision Song Contest, and the Turkish substitution of this entry with a belly dance show, as signs from a distant past irrelevant to progress—"prehistoric"—and not synchronic with Europe. McClintock's term also helps us comprehend these regulatory technologies as manipulation by male forces and capital. If modernity translates into wealth and technological advancement, what remains resistant to modernity is "anachronistic." Therefore, my attachment to these artistic forms had a clearly political meaning since it signified a resistance to maleness and a bourgeois way of constructing the present. Yet this same attachment identified me (and still continues to do so) as an "atavistic and irrational" and somewhat deranged subject.

This work, therefore, is informed by the need to unlearn the rigid and harsh lessons that marked my childhood imagination. I have spent most of my adulthood trying to reconcile and assimilate what my identity as a Greek Cypriot really means; how my masculinity accords this identity and how it remains at odds with it. Even though my answers are not yet adequate, my quest has been productive and replete with telling revelations. My scope, however, is not to secure force and credibility for my arguments through a distinct label that will lock my subjectivity into a particular position. To borrow the words of Smaro Kamboureli, "the pressure I felt to position myself instead of resolving my tensions, kept pointing to various layers of my subjectivity, revealing my identity to be unsettled, continuously disrupted, determined by different alliances on different occasions" (5).[15] Indeed, it is the lack of a specific label that threatened to displace me from the security offered by a certain identification. In fact, the most intriguing quality of my quest is that during its various moments I caught myself obeying the mandates of different voices within me and performing, often with much trepidation, different facets of my personality: the Western-educated "academic," the "dancer," the "queer man," the "Cypriot," the "Greek." In the words of Marta Savigliano, "these voices are my own internal dispute, but far from being a product of my delirious imagination, they speak to me impersonating different audiences of a mixed colonizer/colonized nature" (4).[16]

All these performances take place before the most overwhelming revelations afforded by bodies (including my own) engaged in kinesthetic motion. Dance, with its potential of challenging acceptable postures, may contest the norm and even destabilize an established order. In this subversive sense, the tsifteteli, the Greek version of belly dance, challenges

10

*Introducing
Colonial and
Postcolonial
Dialectics
on the
Subject
of Dance*

the masculine Cypriot body: it configures desire and sensuality and projects this configuration onto a decidedly sexualized posture. I have always been fascinated with the way this particular dance traverses the human body with desire poised on each successive choreographic frame. "[It] focuses on movement of the torso as opposed to movement of the arms and legs as in most Western based forms" (Sellers-Young 141).[17] In my eager gaze, its moves gesture towards an extravagance of impermissible feelings, a certain transgression, and an erotic playfulness. All these mark a defiant contradiction to homosocial dances: the austerely masculine zeibekiko, in its urban solo male form, or the purposely asexual renditions of folkloric community dances such as the kalamatiano, or the "glory" of Greece in the men's tsamiko. The potential for chaos and sexual anarchy seems to lie just within the moves of the tsifteteli as the dance gyrates around the hips, traverses the body in an undulation that concludes with sharp accents, and then descends again on the hips to shimmy unrestrainedly.

What became a significant entry point for me into this project has been my personal investment in examining those agents that have formed the modern Cypriot masculine posture that I have been bequeathed and which proscribes the very movements I have just described. This examination has been crucial in enabling me to comprehend the reasons why belly dance has provided such a powerful means of expression. My exploration, inspired by encounters such as those I quote as epigraphs to this chapter, has led me to the politics of Greek-Turkish relations but has not remained limited to ethnic strife since this dance is interpellated by imperialism and hegemony. Therefore, although Greek-Turkish tensions do not fall within the main province of my investigation, the intricate politics that weave the national issues are quite relevant to British colonialism and Orientalism as well as dance and sexuality.

Colonial Definitions of Acceptable Performance

In Cyprus in the 1960s and '70s the cultural embargo was the result of a climate rife with intense interracial hatred between the Turkish and Greek communities. The tragic events of 1974 that Mariza sang about on the Eurovision Song stage were the military culmination of a cultural and racial civil war. The Greeks of Cyprus felt it was imperative to extricate anything marked as "Eastern," sounds and customs included, since they related to the oppressor. Belly dance itself, which captivated my childhood imagination with its promise for kinesthetic expression, was derided, as was my access to it because of ethnicity and gender. This very denouncement is what makes the tsifteteli a personal site of reconciliation for what my identity as a Greek-Cypriot man interdicts. Within this site, the dance enacts a certain resistance to imperialism (see this chapter's section "Some Notes on the Terms") and reconciliation for the contraries of my Cypriot identity. Therefore, my effort to plot a trajectory through which modern Greek-Cypriot masculinity, as I have inherited and know it, serves a purpose related to the tsifteteli. Various catalysts have constructed this masculinity, complete with its set posture and austere performance. These catalysts are the British colonial administration, the Ottoman conquest preceding it, and modern Greek nationalism.

Cyprus came into British hands in 1878 as part of an economic settlement between the Ottoman Empire and Britain. The spectre of native sexuality was already looming threateningly but also alluringly across the British Empire's horizons, inciting fascination and repulsion—ambivalent responses that are standard in colonial discourse. In Cyprus, the ancient as well as recent past conflated to make legal proscriptions urgent. Before the establishment of British rule, the island was a province of the Ottoman Empire where "spectacular" sexuality enacted itself in practices regarded by Anglo-Saxon bourgeois opinion as lascivious and immoral. Richard Burton's mapping of the "Sotadic Zone" situates the island in the heart of this geographical expanse (with meticulous coordinates) of debauched sexual practices ("Terminal Essay" 206).[18] Apart from Islam, then, Greek myth and ubiquitous archaeological evidence associated the island with Aphrodite's cult, the dissolute and wanton goddess whose worship turned people into sensual and sexually excessive subjects. In fact, according to Burton, Cyprus hosted "one of the head-quarters" of an "androgynic worship" of Aphrodite" ("Terminal Essay" 230-31). Moreover, because dark skin had already become a prime signifier of a subaltern and promiscuous race, the island's population fulfilled the requirements for a racialized erotic and exotic model under the British gaze. "All the Greeks are fond of pleasure," writes Lady Augusta Hamilton, "but the Cypriots give themselves up to a degree of licentiousness, and consider the gratifying of their inclinations as an act of religion" (80).

British administration complicated the tensions in modern Greek Cypriot masculinity through its 1885 legislation on sodomy, the year of the famous Labouchere Amendment to the Criminal Law Amendment

12

*Introducing
Colonial and
Postcolonial
Dialectics
on the
Subject
of Dance*

Act. It deemed acts of gross indecency between men as "misdemeanours" punishable by up to two years of hard labour, thus bringing within the scope of the law all forms of male homosexual activity (Weeks 102). Apart from the politics of foregrounding gender and sexuality and betraying imperial anxiety over sex in the metropolis, this law bears a subtle, albeit powerful, connection to Orientalist discourse, as its sexual anxiety extends to the provinces of the Empire. In *Orientalism* Edward Said has shown how colonial expansion thrived on a discourse that provided the West European metropoles with a way of "knowing" the Orient and maintaining power over it, with discourse as the site where power and knowledge converge. The "Orient," then, is what becomes reified through Western discourse, and not merely for descriptive or identificatory purposes: "Orientalism [is] a Western style for dominating, restructuring, and having authority over the Orient" (3), which stood for the West as "a political vision of reality" (43). British legislation against male homosexuality is an example, to the letter, of Said's argument. The ways in which the British constructed Cyprus and how they determined its rule were largely based on "truths" derived from Western academe's Orientalist inheritance. In fact, Said recognizes "an almost uniform association between the Orient and sex," which he calls "a remarkably persistent motif in Western attitudes to the Orient" (188). Also, in a comment alluding to Foucault's *The History of Sexuality*, he considers it important to establish the fact that "for nineteenth-century Europe, with its increasing *embourgeoisement*, sex had been institutionalized to a very considerable degree" (190). Again, the British law forbidding homosexual acts in the Empire and at home is the result of this institutionalization. Clearly, this act of British legislation functions as a topos where metropolitan politics and peripheral policies merge to discipline and punish.[19]

A discussion of this homophobic legislation lands us directly on the crossroad of (post)colonial politics, gender, race, and sexuality, and, indirectly, dance, since dance is the embodiment and performance of all these.[20] The British law criminalizing sexual acts between adult males constitutes part of the material history of the Cypriot subject's constitution. In terms of imperialism, it is an attack on the culture, ideas, and value systems of the colonized people. To speak in Gayatri Spivak's terms, the British law is one case of "epistemic violence, a complete overhaul of the episteme" (*A Critique of Postcolonial Reason*, 266) that orchestrates the colonized subject's production in the periphery as well as the centre. As a result, the sexual behaviour of the Cypriots, whatever this involved before the British takeover of the island, is forced to comply with Western constructs of heterosexuality and its concomitant homosexuality. Along with sexual behaviour, movement and performance of gender became the manifestations of identity and had to be regulated and curtailed. Finally, discussion of the homophobic legislation and its impact on gender and sexual definition bears important connections with the national struggle against the British occupation. Namely, it relates to how this struggle constructed the Cypriot masculine ideal and what came to be endorsed as "acceptable" behaviour. This struggle was the ultimate test for the implementation of power and change from within the colonized subject and not from without.

The discursive management of sexual practices was produced in tandem with race discourse. For example, Aphrodite, as a phantasm that embodies both archaic and modern sexual excess, does not always mean native dissolution. She is also a classical Greek goddess and revered as such by a West that believed itself to share in the lineage of the Olympic pantheon. The British, therefore, were keen on distinguishing between the "Oriental Turks" and the "Western Greeks." The latter's ties to a classical past were apparent in their dialect, which was the legacy of Homeric Greek. In his autobiographical novel, *Bitter Lemons of Cyprus*, Lawrence Durrell narrates his experience as an English instructor in the public schools of Cyprus in the early 1950s before the Greek-Cypriot uprising against the British. When he assumes a teaching position at the Pancyprian Gymnasium in Nicosia, his class register reminds him of the *Dramatis Personae* in an ancient Greek play with names such as Electra, Io, Chloe, Penelope, and Yiolanthi (130). Significantly, Durrell is careful not to indulge in the same romanticization over boys' names, a gesture that would immediately brand him as a Sotadic lover and thereby denigrate him to the lowest native class. Moreover, there would not be much appeal in a similar litany of Turkish names since, to a Western-educated ear, they do not signify much along the lines of classical splendour.[21] This was the discriminating gaze of the British that played a crucial part in inculcating the Turkish Cypriot and Greek Cypriot ethnic dichotomy in the people's collective imagination.

In the 1955 uprising, which was largely informed by the nationalist ideals inspired by Britain, the Greek Cypriot revolutionaries excluded the Turkish Cypriots and aimed, ultimately, for union (*Enosis*) with Greece, considered to be the mother nation of Greeks in Cyprus. The British worked to suppress the uprising, not only through military means but

14

*Introducing
Colonial and
Postcolonial
Dialectics
on the
Subject
of Dance*

also insidiously, by sowing the seeds of dissension and enmity between the two communities.[22] British policy cultivated Turkish nationalist consciousness as a buffer to Greek nationalism and began to insist that Turkey—not only Greece—should have a say in the future of Cyprus. Under these developments, *Enosis* for the Greeks began to appear an impossible prospect unless the island was partitioned in a way that would satisfy Greece, Turkey, and Britain, the latter maintaining its military bases.[23]

The violence and bloodshed that followed the declaration of the Cyprus Republic resolved none of the serious issues whose settlement was imperative if the island was to become a peaceful and unified state. Atrocities committed by both sides throughout the 1960s have caused wounds that are still bleeding. Greeks and Turks were driven by the conviction that their racial identities were distinct, with differences that justified, even necessitated, an ethnic split. The many centuries during which they coexisted, often in mixed villages and even mixed neighbourhoods, were not catalytic in amalgamating them into one nation, as opposed to hyphenated communities. In fact, these communities did not merely imagine themselves as different segments of the population, but different races for which cohabitation was not a possibility. Despite their declared eagerness to shed their colonized identity, the Greek Cypriot revolutionaries subscribed to the ideological industry of their presumptive Western oppressors. White supremacy seeped into colonized consciousness, creating a bifurcated will: first to be European and "white" and then to assert this superiority over others whom they considered to be of an inferior race, within the same culture. Deeply invested in and proud of their Greek heritage, the Greek Cypriots espoused whiteness and Westernness with great fervour. They had every reason to do so. A certain construction of Greece had been agreed upon by Western European epistemologies to represent the origins of European civilization.[24] Indeed, genuflection to the West bore the expectation of an acceptable identity as well as economic prosperity for modern Cypriots. Moreover, this progress promised also to repair the damages of Cypriot manhood. Usurped by years of Ottoman oppression and British colonial subjugation, Cypriot manhood would rise rejuvenated, victorious, and Western from the flames of the armed uprising.

Already, the parameters of what qualifies as acceptable movement for the Greek Cypriot have begun to set, a process especially active during the decades of anticolonial and intercommunal fighting. By "movement,"

I mean socially appropriate posture and performance of gender and sexuality, as well as the reflection of these in cultural traditions (including dance). The most crucial part in these performances, however, has been played by race and sexuality. Greek Cypriot eagerness to become "European," embedded in the struggle to attain a desired identity, represents a concern over racial identification. Growing up in the 1960s, young Greek Cypriots were exposed to narratives that resounded with imperialist ideologies. Turkish Cypriots were allegedly dark and ugly people devoid of grace and physical charm. In fact, the "handsome" people in the Turkish race were said to be the offspring of Greek women whom Turkish men abducted, raped, or forced into marriage. Such narratives may have retold actual events, yet their processing took place through ideological filters and they circulated as national currency in the collective consciousness. In the words of Ania Loomba, such constructs demonstrate that "religious difference thus became (often rather confusedly) an index of and metaphor for racial, cultural and ethnic differences" (106). Indeed, the construction of the ugly Turk was concomitant with Islam as the religion of the infidel.

And all these religious and cultural prejudices, vivid in the Greek Cypriot imaginary, found expression through sexuality. Certain narratives that strengthened stereotypes became the subject of popular folklore that served as undeniable reminders of Turkish penetration into Greek honour. For example, a Greek woman's rape by a Turkish commander was a recurring narrative. Seen as a form of conquest, rape marks itself on the individual woman's body but also on the body of the nation as a whole, marking with scars that do not heal either on the individual body or on the nation. Benedict Anderson's distinction is useful here: "The fact of the matter is that nationalism thinks in terms of historical destinies, while racism dreams of eternal contaminations, transmitted from the origins of time through an endless sequence of loathsome copulations: outside history" (149). These narratives became invested with a mythopoeic function. They formed the subject of injurious modern myths that Greek Cypriots believed necessary if they were to make sense of their conscious identity in a postcolonial but still imperial state of affairs. Homi Bhabha describes such ideological strategizing quite well:

> In order to understand the productivity of colonial power it is crucial to construct its regime of truth, not to subject its representations to a normalizing judgement. Only then does it become possible to understand the *productive* ambivalence of the object of colonial discourse—that "other-

16

*Introducing
Colonial and
Postcolonial
Dialectics
on the
Subject
of Dance*

ness" which is at once an object of desire and derision, an articulation of difference contained within the fantasy of origin and identity. What such a reading reveals are the boundaries of colonial discourse and it enables a transgression of these limits from the space of that otherness. (67)

Clearly, in these racist constructs the infidel's sexual potency, lasciviousness, cruelty, and abuse loomed large and threatening. Such differences again qualify for identification with Europe and its colonial discourse. Bhabha's arguments on colonial power evoke a relevant dynamic since the constant retelling of these accounts validated a particular "regime of truth." Ministering to this regime was the Greek Cypriot fantasy of origin and identity.

However, the otherness that Turkish Cypriots embodied was not always an object of such a neat contradiction of desire and derision. My own inherited narratives are disparate. Even though my family was directly affected by the intercommunal strife, certain stories of strong friendship between Greeks and Turks survived down to my generation, their survival questioning the absoluteness of this "regime of truth." For example, my grandmother narrated episodes that extolled harmonious relations with Muslim women. She exchanged goods and services with them in a struggle to make ends meet in a poor, agricultural society. Class dynamics, in fact, play an important part in this history. Indeed, Benedict Anderson locates the emergence of racism in class conflicts rather than conflicts between nations:

> The dreams of racism actually have their origin in ideologies of *class*, rather than in those of nation: above all in claims to divinity among rulers and to "blue" or "white" blood and "breeding" among aristocracies. No surprise then that … on the whole, racism and anti-semitism manifest themselves, not across national boundaries, but within them. In other words, they justify not so much foreign wars as domestic repression and domination. (149-50)

His suggestion is particularly poignant in the case of Greek and Turkish Cypriots. Neither community set off to fight an enemy outside the borders of the island. Instead, they fought each other on the neighbouring soil of villages and even in street skirmishes. Although I am not aware of the activities of the elite classes of the island and their role in the conflict, Anderson's analysis has a particularly intriguing application for Cyprus.[25]

From my grandmother and my mother I also learned that my grandfather, Elias (who died in the late 1950s, long before I was born) had close friendships with a number of Turkish men. Apparently, he was also bilingual to a certain extent, but only in spoken language, his bilingualism being a sign of the two communities intermingling.[26] But the narrative that mystifies me the most concerns the musical skill of my male lineage. Apparently, Elias loved to play Turkish and Arabic tunes on his nay, a flute that he carved himself from reeds that he collected from dry river beds.

In the same way that sovereignty maps itself "fully, flatly, and evenly operative over each square centimetre of a legally demarcated territory" (Anderson 19), it also maps itself onto the subject's body. "When it occurs to us, then, to run this question of national definition athwart some already articulated questions of turn-of-the century sexual definition, we must be prepared to look in more directions at once than one," Eve Sedgwick warns (*Tendencies* 150). Retained by the Cypriot republic, the British homophobic legislation that I discuss earlier perpetuates the legacy of colonial rule and makes one wonder how committed Cypriots were to abrogating the oppression of a foreign regime. That the republic kept this law for four decades following its independence is a sad indication that hegemonic structures extend to the Orient, where complex sociocultural processes perpetuate them. Often I indulge in audacious and improper fantasies about my moustached grandfather and his friendships with Turks.[27] Using the language I learned from Sedgwick, I speculate on how these male relationships negotiated the homosocial continuum. Did my grandfather and his friends feel compelled to follow the colonizer's model and repudiate homoeroticism as an element of bonding for a strict homosocial form of domination? Or did their bonds retain some of the character that predated British colonialism—whatever this character may have entailed? While my grandfather played Eastern tunes on his nay, I wonder if he romanticized the melodies and if he imagined a male or a female body interpreting the moves. And how did he embody these melodies at weddings and religious festivals? In what ways did his hips articulate the music or did his masculine posture remain firm? I pose these questions because there is something subversive in the very exercise. In Cypriot tradition, masculine posture is to be accepted and revered—not profaned by interpretation such as the one I attempt here. I wish, however, to challenge the complacency and test the brittle balance of masculinity through epistemic gestures. My dance attempts the same.

18

*Introducing
Colonial and
Postcolonial
Dialectics
on the
Subject
of Dance*

Performing Theory

The history, or rather histories, that I have attempted to outline here are
crucial in providing the context in which my body registers its presence
in this project. In this endeavour I occupy the position of reader as much
as writer since I do not feel represented by the production of contemporary political discourse on the "Cyprus problem" and issues of ethnicity
and national identity. Therefore, I voyage across the landscape of memory, my body asking questions about the fugitive nature of my performance as well as that of others. I imagine my itinerary as similar to that
planned for the reader of *Corporealities*:

> Voyaging across the landscape that memory provides, the reader is asked
> to revel in and take inspiration from the fugitive nature of any perform-
> ance. Travelling to the ethnographic field and then to the historical
> archive, the reader winds, hurtles, and backtracks, or zooms along tra-
> jectories that attempt to account for the pasts and presents that make up
> the interpretation and representation of past movement. (Foster xvi)

In the process of mapping a historical trajectory of Cypriot masculinity I
am, in effect, attempting to assess my own masculinity and, thereby, assess
alternative performances of identity, both sexual and national, in an effort
to disrupt colonialist construction. I also need to study ways in which
these catalysts—British imperialism, Ottoman conquest, and Greek
nationalism—interacted with my personal adorations, namely my passionate investment in Mariza Koch and belly dance. This investment
represented a cathexis in art, promising to express, mend, and reconcile.
I am grateful to these apocryphal passions because they formulated my
personal mythology that shaped the particularities of my individual "masculinity" within Cypriot culture.

A scene from Anna Kokkinos's Greek-Australian film *Head On*
(1998), based on the novel *Loaded* by Christos Tsiolkas, presents a characteristic and somewhat humorous illustration of the traumatic impact
of the Greek-Turkish conflict. In a scene that combines issues of sexuality and gender performance and, later, dances in the Greek club, "The
Steki," the film exposes the issues I try to explore here. Toula and Ari, the
two main characters whose Greek ethnicity is a pivotal marker in the
film and the novel, enter a taxi whose driver turns out to be Turkish.
Toula, whose female drag becomes critical at this moment, turns to the
taxi driver to announce: "Your great grandfather raped my great grandmother." There is an outburst of laughter from both her and Ari follow-

ing her comment, which, paradoxically, bonds them with the Turkish driver. He turns out to be left wing, well informed, and sensitive in his determinations on the recent history of Greece and Turkey (he has a tape of Manos Loizos's song "O Dromos," a song that derives from a left-wing musical tradition and would be identified as such by most Greeks watching the film). This exchange evokes humour as it parodies cultural memory with its reliance on trauma and drama for its impact and circulation. Such turns make this particular encounter a rare and special moment that questions the enmity between Greeks and Turks as a deeply rooted and ineradicable division, as official culture would have it. Ultimately, I find the scene vindicates awareness, reflection, and critique when considering the political and cultural relations between the two countries and their people.

That both Greek-Australian characters, Toula and Ari, are queer is also critical in this analysis, since their transgressive sexuality is what drives the incisive critique that the film makes. In fact, their sexuality and especially Toula's in-drag, feminine performance, mark the body in ways that carry the attributes of dance. Drag as gender performativity, along with alternative sexual identities, pushes the physical demarcations of the body in its quest for artistic utterances, which are political by extension. As it materializes on the human body, dance performs similar functions, including the questioning in Fanon's invocation, "Oh my body, make of me always a man who questions!" (232). It is, of course, quite significant that when Toula appears at "The Steki" what she performs, in response to the awkward and uncomfortable reception by the crowd, is a tsifteteli—a performance that aligns her at this moment with the tradition of transvestite dancers that I will be discussing in chapter 3. The Greek club is the establishment in the film (and the novel) where all the "glamour," "glory," and social oppression suffered by virtue of being "Greek" in Australia enact themselves eloquently through the most representative Greek popular dances.

My efforts, however, do not aspire to unearth pristine, unspoiled forms of dance or arcane kinesthetic texts that await discovery. I mean to decolonize, following Marta Savigliano's assertion that "decolonization means rejecting the search for the origins and authenticity of the colonized in order to concentrate on the specific, original, and authentic ways in which imperialism operates" (9). There is no tsifteteli to perform that is not colonized. I do not seek to emulate a quest for origins and authenticity (such a search is Dora Stratou's main concern as I discuss

20

Introducing
Colonial and
Postcolonial
Dialectics
on the
Subject
of Dance

in the final chapter), and I cannot refurbish an unspoiled or "authentic" rendition of this dance. This does not mean erasing, defacing, or exploiting it mercilessly but exploring the complex struggles through which it has survived down to me and through which it has afforded me a means of expression and deliverance. Savigliano's comment on tango is an apt expression of my aspiration: "tangoing through postmodernity I perform my awkward decolonizing kicks in the midst of that patriarchal and colonial dance. There are no other dances available for me" (227). In a similar process, I sway my hips, relying on their articulations to perform counter readings to patriarchy and coloniality.

As I attempt to decipher the inscriptions of my position, I am confident that the historiographies I explore in the chapters that follow connect with my own. I research with a corporeal investment and with the conviction that to explore the space I occupy, the position into which I have been written, as Spivak puts it, is a crucial step towards recognizing the visceral impacts of colonialism and postcolonialism. Therefore, even though some of the chapters might appear to have distinct historical and thematic foci, they are all written in a manner that relies on both "centrifugal and centripetal" movements (terms I borrow from Smaro Kamboureli): I focus closely on dancing bodies and deploy their motion to disentangle the web of ideological implications of movement as a primary social text. These implications weave gender, race, class, and imperialism into complex hybrid patterns. I use "hybrid" as Robert Young explores it in *Colonial Desire*, where it suggests contamination and impurity.

In the process of examining various imperial texts, I have repeatedly encountered a certain eagerness on the part of the subjects producing these texts to surrender to the seduction of the body performing Middle Eastern dance. In fact, the imperial subject often seems prepared to go beyond seduction. It seems eager to cross the threshold of anachronistic space and abandon itself to the fantasy of embodying the dance in order to experience the metamorphosis that movement may afford. Thus, Middle Eastern dance offers that space where transformation is possible but is curtailed by the perils that such deviation may engender, perils that are intrinsic in the process of transformation. What I argue is that this dance is derided and adored precisely because of its ambivalent construction. This profound ambivalence is what marks the typological relationship of Middle Eastern performer and the Western spectator's gaze. In Homi Bhabha's use of the term, such ambivalence becomes an essential province of investigation in colonial dynamics. Bhabha's analysis focuses not on the object of the gaze but on how the gaze is staged at the psychic level, hence the contiguous relationship between ambivalence, fetish, and stereotype, both of which operate through scopophilia (i.e., the pleasure of looking):

> The fetish or stereotype gives access to an "identity" which is predicated as much on mastery and pleasure as it is on anxiety and defence, for it is a form of multiple and contradictory belief in its recognition of difference and disavowal of it. This conflict of pleasure/unpleasure, mastery/defence, knowledge/disavowal, absence/presence, has a fundamental significance for colonial discourse. For the scene of fetishism is also the scene of the reactivation and repetition of primal fantasy—the subject's desire for a pure origin that is always threatened by its division, for the subject must be gendered to be engendered, to be spoken. (75)

Bhabha's deployment of these terms is particularly useful in an examination of dance since they emphasize "the mutualities and negotiations across the colonial divide" (Moore-Gilbert 116), and this is the kind of interaction and dynamic that performance evokes. In fact, there will be further need to revisit Bhabha's analysis in the course of this project (I return to the above quotation in the following chapter), since discussions of "exoticized" performance benefit greatly from the paradoxical schemata of desire and disavowal. According to Robert Young, Bhabha has made "ambivalence the constitutive heart of his analyses ... in which the periphery—the borderline, the marginal, the unclassifiable, the doubtful—has become the equivocal, indefinite, indeterminate ambivalence that characterizes the centre" (*Colonial Desire* 161). This "political reversal at a conceptual level," as Young calls it (161), precisely sums up the effect of Oriental dance on the metropolitan centre: this dance is the equivocal, colonial practice that transfers itself into the very heart of the imperial metropolis—a site that I am using here as metaphor for an ideological core—causing the centre to shimmer before the vision of outlandish and delectable possibilities.

Nonetheless, I have resisted making Bhabha's discourse the foundation of my examination partly because I did not wish to fix my observations on performance, colonialism, and sexuality onto one specific discursive formula. Anne McClintock's critique of ambivalence is useful here. While she acknowledges the value and importance of Bhabha's contribution, she is also concerned about the efficacy of agency in the theory of ambivalence:

22

*Introducing
Colonial and
Postcolonial
Dialectics
on the
Subject
of Dance*

Locating agency in ambivalence runs the risk of what can be called a
fetishism of form: the projection of historical agency onto formal abstractions that are anthropomorphized and given a life of their own. Here
abstractions become historical actors; discourse desires, dreams and does
the work of colonialism while also ensuring its demise. In the process,
social relations between humans appear to metamorphize into struc-
tural relations between forms—through a formalist fetishism that effectively elides the messier questions of historical change and social activism.
(63-64)

My interest extends beyond establishing set modalities. As this introduction indicates, I wish to engage with the economy of passion implicit in
any relationship with dance, as well as with the effects of colonialism on
social, racial, and national dynamics.[28] My *Dramatis Personae* aspires to
cast not merely abstractions but movement as well. In its physicality,
dance is a unique tool in such exploration because it appeals to the body
itself, the site of vital performances. Indeed, what I am investigating is a
colonialist dynamic that constantly shifts in a dance that is literal but
also metaphorical. Gender and sexuality are also shifting values, hence
the ambivalence and the crisis they incite. "If," as McClintock points
out, "all discourses are ambivalent, what distinguishes the discourse of the
empowered from the discourse of the disempowered?" (64). While developing the histories that I am concerned with, I am evoking the tense
structures of the privileged and the unprivileged, the imperial subject
and the native, or, in McClintock's terms, the empowered and the disempowered. As Anne McClintock reminds us, I need, therefore, to locate
ambivalence not in all discourses, but in particular desires and particular moments that involve dance.

Another obstacle to using Homi Bhabha is the way he elides gender
difference, thus implicitly ratifying gender power, "so that masculinity
becomes the invisible norm of postcolonial discourse" (McClintock 64-
65). To a certain extent, the authority of this masculine posture impedes
my engagement with Bhabha's discourse. Instead, more aligned with my
theoretical aspirations is Jill Dolan's approach to theory and its role in her
life and work:

Through theory I can articulate the roots of my own identity in the conflicting discourses of lesbianism and Judaism and know that there is no
comfortable place for me within any single discourse. Theory enables me
to describe the differences within me and around me without forcing me
to rank my allegiances or my oppressions. As feminist critic Gayle Austin

would say, theory enables the divided subject to fall into the cracks of difference and to theorize productively from there, knowing that truth is changeable, permeable, and, finally, irrelevant. (95)

Robert Young's comments on "truth" complement Dolan's position: "truth, like historicity, is derived from particular discursive practices; it operates internally as a form of regulation, as well as being the historical product of the battle between different discursive regimes" (*White Mythologies* 70). Apart from offering an outlet to my bind over "truth," Dolan also privileges sexuality and religious background in her approach. In her circumscription, Dolan moves along the same parameters that I need to explore, difference and subject division, helping me situate my goals and myself theoretically.

I work on dance yet refrain from providing a working definition of it. Paradoxically, I feel more secure in the indeterminacy of the term because my intentions are devious (in the etymological sense of the term): I intend to move in and out of dance's formal representations because the performances I would like to track also concern gender, race, and ethnic identity. Therefore, while on the one hand, I am writing about dance performances which are formal in that they are arranged, staged, and with an audience and often some sort of an economic exchange, I also hope to escape with occasional excursions into performances in which the body confirms its often varying sexual, gender, and racial allegiances through movement. Thus, I feel motivated by a certain empathy with the figures I discuss, while spatial, ideological, and temporal distances seriously qualify this empathy. In an ambitious attempt to facilitate my discourse and negotiate my performances, I "choreograph" my writing by occasionally interpolating my text with sections on my private, almost unrehearsed, acts of personal events and raw memories. I need this performance if I am to comprehend the space I occupy and its historical explication. Thus, my effort is to choreograph theory and theorize choreography, performing dance in the medium of the written word. This "staging of writing," as Susan Leigh Foster would call it, aspires to recreate the dance as it summons up the rhythm or dynamics and structure of the event, so it provides an analogous experience for the reader as the dance performance does for the viewer.[29]

Also significant in my analysis on performers (both male and female) are the implications of travel on European influence and imperial expansion. In the context of nineteenth- and early twentieth-century imperialism, Europeanization was not the job of merely governments and states.

24

*Introducing
Colonial and
Postcolonial
Dialectics
on the
Subject
of Dance*

Each travel itinerary of hordes of merchants, missionaries, and adventurers who permeated the non-European world inscribed, in some small but nevertheless important way, the features of European expansionism. A glance at Amelia Edwards's travel narrative from Egypt, 1873, gives some idea of the volume of Western human traffic and the magnitude of its impact. Staying at Shepheard's Hotel in Cairo, she depicts the crowd of guests as follows:

> Here assemble daily some two to three hundred persons of all ranks, nationalities, and pursuits; half of whom are Anglo-Indians homeward or outward bound, European residents, or visitors established in Cairo for the winter. The other half, it may be taken for granted, are going up the Nile.... Nine-tenths of those whom [the newcomer] is likely to meet up the river are English or American. The rest will be mostly German, with a sprinkling of Belgian and French. So far *en bloc*; but the details are more heterogeneous still. Here are invalids in search of health; artists in search of subjects; sportsmen keen upon crocodiles; statesmen out for a holiday; special correspondents alert for gossip; collectors on the scent of papyri and mummies; men of science with only scientific ends in view; and the usual surplus of idlers who travel for the mere love of travel or the satisfaction of a purposeless curiosity. (1-2)

Each of these travellers that Edwards describes has played their individual part as agents of colonial domination. Gayatri Spivak incisively theorizes the process through which such a scripting of the colony took place through each body that journeyed through that space. There was no "innocuous" itinerary. A British soldier's wanderings through the Indian landscape contribute to the "worlding" of the colonized land. (I discuss the term further as well as its relevance to my project in the conclusion to chapter 5.)

The traffic of ordinary European travellers, explorers, missionaries, fortune hunters, and settlers that Edwards describes, and Spivak's theory of the way they inscribed the foreign land, are significant in my examination of dance. In the same way that these travellers inscribed the land, they also inscribed the dancing body, interpreting it for the Empire but also reinterpreting it to the native as well. This process of reinscription and reinterpretation forms an essential component of my project. Furthermore, I work with the confidence that while undergoing this "Europeanization," the dancer and the viewer set up an economy that involves, but is not limited to, the satisfaction of mutual needs. In their intercourse they enter what at times resembles a wrestling, a grappling to impose their power over each other, and at other times resembles a scopic intercourse that consumes both performer and imperial subject with longing. Ultimately, however, the uninitiated and phobic Western viewer is most at home with the dancer as a threatening image. Constructed in terms of threat, the dancer yields the art to a colonial order, thereby absolving the subject of the deviant transformations that Middle Eastern dance suggests.

Some Notes on the Terms

Few moments caused me as much discomfort in this project—while also highlighting the complexity of the issues that I deal with—as the attempt to provide a glossary. An explication of the nomenclature would be a polite and also necessary gesture to my readers, yet it makes me uneasy since the terms themselves are fluid. In fact, despite my experience with them, they still remain in a sense unknown, thus making me realize I am hardly the authority to decide upon and provide definitions. The terms I work with are, in some cases, unsatisfactory because of their problematic and complex history. However, the attempted definitions are an important requirement for these very same reasons.

In my text I have decided not to italicize either the various terms used for this particular dance idiom or the names of musical instruments. My decision is political since it relates to English as an imperial language and my reluctance to evoke the terms' foreignness and force them into italicized margins each time they appear.

Belly Dance Nomenclature

To begin with, *belly dance, danse du ventre, Middle Eastern dance, Oriental dance,* and *tsifteteli* are signifiers that refer to widely varying interpretations of a related dance idiom. In their representation of hybrid art forms, all these terms are, however, fraught with political problems that are quite telling in themselves. *Belly dance,* for example, relays a sad history since, along with *danse du ventre,* it evokes the immersion of an art form into a Western culture and its absorption into a male heterosexist discourse. *Danse du ventre* denotes the French colonial conquest of Algeria and Tunisia as well as other regions of the Middle East, so it is redolent with imperial soldiers' heterosexual pursuit of hedonist fulfillment on colonized subjects' bodies. Such pursuit is what motivated the printing of postcards that Malek Alloula makes the subject of his anticolonial

Introducing
Colonial and
Postcolonial
Dialectics
on the
Subject
of Dance

project *The Colonial Harem*. With regards to *Oriental dance*, this seems to be one of those interesting paradigms that conflate auto-exoticization and colonial dynamics. The English term is a translation of the Arabic *Raqs Sharqi*, or "Dance of the East," the Arabic term indicating that in the Arab world, especially in Egypt, this is a dance of the "East." This designation may result from an Arabic adoption of the European identification "Dance of the East" (also "Ανατολίτικος Χορός" in Greek), since this was the most widely experienced form of native dance in cafés frequented by Westerners who referred to it as such (Stone 35). Cassandra Lorius notes that *Raqs Sharqi* and *belly dance* have come to be used interchangeably and both derive from *danse du ventre* of the early Orientalists. "Belly dance," she writes, "has become part of a Hollywood stereotype conjuring up notions of exoticism and eroticism. The appropriation of Egyptian dance by cultural colonialism has had a significant impact on Egyptian dance, which has further adapted to the cabaret setting of the nightclub, introduced to Egypt in the 1920s" (298, n4). (Hollywood Orientalism is a theme that Rebecca Stone develops in "Cinematic Salomés.") Moreover, conducting research among members of the diasporic Egyptian community in Toronto, Kathleen Fraser found that most of her informants were happy with the term *Raqs Baladi*, Baladi being a rich and important signifier in Arabic since it implies a number of precious values that include "folk," "authentic," "traditional," "down-to-earth," and "village" as well as *belly dance* ("The Aesthetics of Belly Dance" 43-47). Magda Saleh, dance scholar and an authority on Egyptian folklore traditions, tells us that in Egypt the most common terms for this dance are *Raqs Baladi*, *Raqs Sharqi*, *Raqs Arabi*, and *Raqs Masri*, the latter word being the Arabic name of "Egypt" (128). I find this last term extremely interesting since using the nation's name to label a certain dance might reveal the extent of its popularity and representation of Egypt itself.

Furthermore, *Middle Eastern dance* is a vague location and as a term too reliant on a geographical area almost as arbitrarily defined as Richard Burton's the "Sotadic Zone," a reproduction of an Orientalist fantasy fixed temporally and spatially. Moreover, *Middle East* is "a term of Western military provenance" (Stokes and Davis 255), a provenance that recalls violence since the division of Cyprus and its identity crises are intricately connected to the term and its postcolonial denotations. In recent international politics, the "strategic location" of Cyprus has provoked British, American, Greek, and Turkish interests and has directed their decision making about the future of the island. And, juxtaposed with these politics is that eager aspiration of Cypriots to be "European." Therefore, the term is a potent signifier. It refers to a landscape that I am strongly attached to, a confused but rich culture that straddles East and West, and a deplorable political situation that has led to horror and devastation.[30] Yet, "Middle East" does not evoke only the Cyprus problem. In fact, for most people in the West it evokes the Palestinian-Israeli conflict and the West's role in upholding the tension in the area. Since 2002, violence in the West Bank has escalated into the worst conflicts in the last decades, with Israeli forces increasing their military operations. In doing so they perpetuate a conflict that is the direct outcome of European colonization in the area.

Using the terms for this dance has been a process of constant negotiation and of risk taking, a trying exercise that constantly tested my own acceptance and prejudices. I dislike *belly dance* because of the responses (smirk, sarcasm, derision) it generally solicits, yet I use it because it is familiar, and because respectful usage might reclaim it to a certain extent. In relation to the Greek version, I use *tsifteteli* to distinguish it from modern Egyptian renditions which I refer to mostly as Oriental dance. The terms could also engender some misunderstanding that may arise from this project. I realize that, just as Edward Said has been criticized for a monolithic representation of the East, I may be criticized for imposing homogeneity upon a variety of different dance traditions. What Kuchuk Hanem (see chapter 2) danced was not *tsifteteli* and it was not *belly dancing* either (Derek Gregory makes the anachronistic error of referring to the *ghawazee* as *belly dancers* [143]). Similarly, Azizeh's rendition, which appears to have been rather different from Kuchuk's, was neither. And yet, both performed, mostly solo, a dance whose idiom—elaborate hip articulations, isolations, movement on the vertical and horizontal axis but not across large space—is clearly related. I use *belly dance* and *Oriental dance* often interchangeably while I reserve *Middle Eastern dance* for the moments when I hope to obtain a more general context for my argument (hence its appointment in the subtitle of this book). Shifting from one to the other is sometimes not so much an attempt at precision as a visitation of all the different sites where these terms transport us.

Moreover, the appellations for dancers have an equivocal cultural stance in Arabic and Turkish. *Khawals*, for example, is the Arabic plural term for male dancers. They had colleagues, the *Gink*, who were "generally," Edward W. Lane qualifies, Jewish, Armenian, and Greek, as well as Turkish (389). Stephen Murray notes that if it were not for the qual-

28

Introducing
Colonial and
Postcolonial
Dialectics
on the
Subject
of Dance

ifier "generally," he would interpret Lane's distinction between Khawal and Gink as ethnic. However, Murray suggests that the distinction may "differentiate explicitness of availability for sexual hire rather than shared 'tribal' background" (46, n24). In Turkey, male performers were known as *koçek*. According to some sources (Thijs Janssen's main source is Jakob Salomo Bartholdy who wrote in the early nineteenth century), the ethnicity of this class of male performers in the Ottoman Empire was made up again mostly of Greeks, Armenians, and Jews, since a Turkish man would not deign to be a public performer (Janssen 84).[31] Today, the linguistic development of these terms tells of colonialism and the way it has constructed homosexuality, not as an act but as a lifestyle with an attached identity. In both Turkey and Egypt, at least, the names once used for male dancers now signify homosexuals. In Arabic *khawal* is clearly a reference to a gay man and in contemporary Turkey a *koçek* covers "both transvestites and transsexuals" (Janssen 83).

Similarly, *ghawazee*, the general term by which female dancers were known in Egypt during most of the nineteenth century, has now become derogatory as it implies an infamous and dishonourable woman of questionable morality, as Karen van Nieuwkerk explains in her ethnographic study, "A Trade Like Any Other": Female Singers and Dancers in Egypt (1-8). Providing explications for the origins or etymologies of the term *ghawazee* has been an assignment favoured by many researchers on Middle Eastern dance. Leona Wood informs us that the term appears after the advent of Islam and "its apparent etymology from the Arabic *ghawa: to be enamoured* seems to make it an appropriate appellation rather than, as has been repeatedly asserted, the name of a special tribe."[32] Writing in 1989, Wendy Buonaventura disregards Wood's suggestion and insists unequivocally that "the original *ghawazee* were gypsies, though the word has come to be used as a generic term for dancers rather than to denote a particular tribe, or tribes, as was once the case" (39). To complicate matters even more, the term *almeh* (plural *awâlim*) seems to have become an adopted name for dancers, once the *ghawazee* began to be subject to legislative constraints.

The *Awâlim* were learned female singers who enjoyed great respect since their singing perpetuated an old oral tradition. Alain Weber believes them to serve as the "living repositories of the ancient qayna, the slave singers of pre-Islamic times."[33] Apparently, they sang behind a wooden lattice so they would not be visible, a custom that draws attention to visibility as engendering contamination. Aurality, on the other hand, classifies as a noble sense. Since the conflation of the two names might be related to Mohamed Ali's prohibition in 1834, which forced *ghawazee* to claim they were *awâlim* so as to escape banishment (see chapter 3), and with European demand for their services increasing, then the confusion over *awâlim* and *ghawazee* might also have relevant and interesting colonial underpinnings. Gustave Flaubert's sarcastic remark to Louis Bouilhet gestures towards imperial condescension: "the word *almeh* means 'learned woman,' 'blue stocking,' or 'whore'—which proves, Monsieur, that in all countries women of letters ...!!!" (Steegmuller, *Flaubert in Egypt* 129). In an article on the famous Egyptian dancer Tahia Carioca, Edward Said identifies this much-respected and beloved dancer as an artist who revived this tradition:

> This was the all-but-forgotten role of *almeh* (literally, a learned woman), spoken of by nineteenth-century European visitors to the Orient such as Edward Lane and Flaubert. The *almeh* was a courtesan of sorts, but a woman of significant accomplishments. Dancing was only one of her gifts; others were the ability to sing and recite classical poetry, to discourse wittily, to be sought after for her company by men of law, politics, and literature. ("Homage to a Belly-Dancer" 350)

Anthony Shay, however, disagrees that the *almeh* "socialized with and made learned conversation with their patrons." Rather, he believes them to be experts in their craft, able to memorize enormous amounts of poetry and music to perform, but not intellectual thinkers who mixed with men. The *almeh* (*awâlim*) were vocalists who may have occasionally danced, while the *ghawazee* were generally dancers. "The specialization that we attribute to them is a Western division of labour that did not match the actual performance activities of these performers" (personal mail, 6 Feb. 2002).

Kohl

This is the word for eye makeup in a number of Eastern languages. Its application has always been a ubiquitous practice, vital for its aesthetic and medicinal purposes both in antiquity and in recent times. That the application of kohl has had "beneficial" qualities widens the theoretical angles of perception. In hot, sunny regions it provided physical relief when applied to tired eyes by producing a cooling and soothing effect. Richard Burton, who is known to have exaggerated or sensationalized some of his descriptions and explications of Eastern habits and customs, "found this powder a great preservative from ophthalmia in desert-trav-

30

Introducing
Colonial and
Postcolonial
Dialectics
on the
Subject
of Dance

elling" (Burton, "Supplement" 11, n11). Kohl was applied to allay the effects of heat as well as to function as a pre-industrial kind of sunglasses with no lenses. For Orientalists, however, to acknowledge such uses required a necessary revision of imperial standardized notions of beauty that had been constructed without any regard to world climatology.

In a dance context, kohl's intervention in the natural landscape of the face assumes a remarkable performativity conjuring a host of meanings and significations. In his book *Sacred Prostitution*, which examines the institution of religious prostitution in the ancient Near East, the Greek scholar Andreas Lentakis refers to a myth from Pausanias that involves Alfeios and the goddess Artemis. Alfeios was enamoured of the goddess and pursued her to Letrinous where she was presiding in a nocturnal rite with her female attendants. Foreseeing the danger imminent in his advances—apparently Alfeios's intention was to rape her—the goddess escaped recognition by applying a layer of mud over her face. Thus, by resorting to masquerade she protected herself as well as her attendants and evaded the threat posed by an undesirable male pursuer. Lentakis draws attention to the myth's initiatory character and further points out that makeup and masquerade seem to have played significant roles in initiation rituals, not only in mainland Greece but also in a number of worship sites found all over the Middle East of antiquity (242-43). This myth is valuable for its understanding of makeup as a narrative of concealment through transformation, a concept that is crucial to dance as mystery.

In connection with colonialism and Middle Eastern dance in particular, makeup has always been an inexhaustible source of fascination in Western travellers, and this fascination is closely related to their perceptions of dance in a number of ways. Ultimately, my discussion of kohl wants to theorize some of the intense implications of ornamentation and makeup in Oriental dance by tracing the thickly delineated contours of seduction drawn by instruments of adornment. These inscribe a cyclical trajectory in the imperialist gaze as instruments of subordination that transform into allure. I will begin this exploration of makeup's strong appeal by revisiting some of the annotations that Edward Lane, Richard Burton, and Henry Torrens wrote in order to explicate kohl in their versions of *The Arabian Nights*.[34] Edward Lane volunteers a variety of interesting details on the preparation and uses for kohl:

> Kohl is a black powder, with which most of the Arab and many other women blacken the edges of the eyelids. The most common kind is the

smoke-black which is produced by burning a kind of frankincense. An inferior kind is the smoke-black produced by burning the shells of almonds. These are believed to be beneficial to the eyes, but are generally used merely for the sake of ornament. Among other kinds which are particularly employed for their beneficial effect upon the eye are several ores of lead, reduced to a fine powder. Antimony is said to have been, in former times, the most esteemed kind of kohl. The powder is applied by means of a small probe of wood, ivory, or silver, the end of which is moistened, and then dipped in the powder, and drawn along the edges of the eyelids (Burton, "Supplement" 12, n21).

Torrens (1806-1852), whose translation is a landmark in the history of westernization of the *Arabian Nights*, also comments on eye makeup in the East: "the use of various descriptions of dark pigment round the eyelids is a very common Eastern custom; it is supposed to increase their lustre and to strengthen the sight, and is looked upon as a great embellishment to the countenance" (Burton, "Supplement" 11, n11). Richard Burton, who sees it as his duty to enlighten his readers with the help of lavish illustrations, seems quite taken by the various procedures that makeup involves. His fascination is evident in his effort to explain to his readers how makeup is applied, and in the details that he relates: "The powder is kept in an étui called Makhalah and applied with a thick blunt needle to the inside of the eyelid, drawing it along the rim" (Burton, "Supplement" 11, n11). Like Lane, Burton is eager to provide plenty of detail, an eagerness that betrays a certain fascination and rapture in the activity.[35] In both descriptions there is an almost campy interest in the objects and the artistry that is obviously involved and an envious recognition of this artistry which is manifest in the nature of the descriptions: "drawn along the edges of the eyelids" (Lane) and "drawing it along the rim" (Burton).[36] I am suggesting, therefore, that these men nurtured such a fascination for makeup ritual that kohl becomes a fetish of sorts, something that needs to be conquered and at the same time yielded to. In this way, kohl is analogous to dance, which is also caught in this cycle of "becomings."

Finally, narcissism and a certain kind of auto-eroticism form an integral part of the makeup ritual. The moment when the male or female dancer bends before the mirror to apply kohl is endowed with a certain mysticism. It is a moment of self-devotion and self-absorption. To elaborate further on the significance of narcissistic and voyeuristic themes, I would like to draw from Teresa de Lauretis's comments on the "tropical"—as she calls it—question "How do I look?":

32

Introducing
Colonial and
Postcolonial
Dialectics
on the
Subject
of Dance

The first take is to hear it narcissistically (why not? I am, after all, female and queer), to hear it as an intransitive verb: how do I look—to you, to myself, how do I appear, how am I seen? What are the ways in which I'm seen or can be seen, the conditions of my visibility? The second take is to hear the transitive, active verb, subject to object: how do I look at you, at her, at the film, at myself? How do I see, what are the modes, constraints, and possibilities of my seeing, the terms of vision for me? The next take is to hear the verb as active but not transitive: how do I look *on*, as the film unrolls from reel to reel in the projector, as the images appear and the story unfolds on the screen, as the fantasy scenario unveils and the soundtrack plays on in my head? (223)

The look of made-up eyes is relevant to some of these important questions de Lauretis raises. Strangely, kohl also "frames" the eyes in a literal and tropical way. The literal is fairly straightforward as it implies a shadow on the eyelid or a line that traces the rim of the eye. This physical aspect affects the viewer in the way he sees and thereby influences by this gaze the conditions of the woman's visibility. However, apart from being a physical demarcation of the eye, it is also a demarcation of the woman's perception since when we look at a picture the frame around it is just as important and just as much a part of the picture itself. What I am saying is that the frame exists not only for the viewer who can clearly discern its physical demarcation but also for the woman looking through made-up eyes. This physical frame is not within her field of vision but forms instead, the frame through which the subject observes her world. Frame, in this case, does not suggest restriction or confinement; rather, an expansion of the art of gazing transitively and intransitively.

Postcolonial, Neo-colonial

Finally, I turn to some contested terms that are fundamental in my approach. Again, I do not hope to explicate these terms adequately or definitively. Instead, I wish to acknowledge their complexity and indicate how I employ them but also the process through which I try to derive meaning from their constantly shifting form.

Anne McClintock resists the singular, monolithic nature of the term *postcolonial*, used ahistorically and according to the nineteenth-century image of linear progress. As a result, she finds that *postcolonial*, although heralding the end of a historical era, "reorients the globe once more around a single, binary opposition: colonial-postcolonial" (10). Moreover, she argues that postcolonial *theory* is a singular term that recentres global history around the single rubric of European time so that "colonialism returns at the moment of its disappearance" (11). Ella Shohat also expresses concern over the term's temporal and spatial placement. Shohat finds, however, that "the term *neocolonialism* usefully designates broad relations of geoeconomic hegemony. When examined in relation to *neocolonialism*, the term *postcolonial* undermines a critique of contemporary colonialist structures of domination, more available through the repetition and revival of the *neo*" (134). Shohat calls for historical, geopolitical, and cultural interrogation and contextualization of the *postcolonial*, since "each frame illuminates only partial aspects of systemic modes of domination, of overlapping collective identities, and of contemporary global relations" (138).

In my usage, I assign *neocolonial* to the recent dominating attitudes prevalent in systems but also in individuals who succumb to superpower ideologies. As for the *postcolonial*, I have never experienced it, since, as a citizen of Cyprus, I have never moved beyond the *post* of *colonialism*. Britain maintains bases on the island, referred to as "Sovereign Base Areas," while the events of 1974 secured the partition of Cyprus. I live in a divided city where the recent ease of restrictions in movement between north and south has served to emphasize the separation and distance between Greek and Turkish Cypriots.[37] In this state of affairs, and with successive Cypriot governments being obstinate and oppressive in different ways and subject to the relentless tyranny of the Church, there is not much independence, "freedom," or *postcoloniality* left to celebrate. My body, along with my island, remains colonized.

Colonialism and Imperialism

In certain instances, by employing the term *colonial* I do not refer to historical fact. Egypt in the 1850s, for example, was not the colony of a European power but a province of the Ottoman Empire. Similarly, Greece has never been administered as a European colony, only a British protectorate following the Second World War. However, Greece is still subject to imperialism. For example, the Eurovision Song Contest can be seen as an imperial endeavour where a number of metropolitan centres converge in an event that affects certain uncolonized European countries that do not rate highly on the "European-meaning-civilized" index. In my usage of the terms *imperial* and *colonial*, I am aware that I deviate from the denotative meanings of these terms and that such deviation involves certain risks. As Ania Loomba encouragingly points out, how-

34

Introducing
Colonial and
Postcolonial
Dialectics
on the
Subject
of Dance

ever, *colonialism* and *imperialism* are concepts difficult to pin down to a single semantic meaning and are easier understood by relating their shifting meanings to historical processes (4). In other words, the terms themselves are absorbed into their own elusive dance. Nevertheless, what I refer to with the term *colonialism* are the effects and influences of imperial domination, not only on geographical sites, bodies of land and water but on human bodies as well. When it comes to distinguishing between the terms *colonialism* and *imperialism*, I am following Loomba who suggests that

> one useful way ... might be to not separate them in temporal but in spatial terms and to think of imperialism or neo-imperialism as the phenomenon that originates in the metropolis, the process which leads to domination and control. Its result, or what happens in the colonies as a consequence of imperial domination is colonialism or neo-colonialism. Thus the imperial country is the "metropole" from which power flows, and the colony or neo colony is the place which it penetrates and controls. Imperialism can function without formal colonies (as in the United States imperialism today) but colonialism cannot. (6-7)

Imperialism, then, here refers to that discourse which affirmed the global centrality of the West and its assumptions concerning civilization, technological advancement, language, and so on. As Anne McClintock defines them, the three governing themes of Western imperialism are "the transmission of white, male power through control of colonized women; the emergence of a new global order of cultural knowledge; and the imperial command of commodity capital" (1-3). As I argue, the colony also shares a form of kinesthetic power in this economy of penetration and control, as its dance traditions respond to the emerging global order of cultural knowledge. *Imperialism* conjures images of social superiority and imposition on the Other—the Middle Eastern Other, in this context—while also drawing attention to the complex dynamics that dominated the West's witnessing of cultural production in the East. Finally, the term *colonial* is useful in corporeal terms as it denotes the process that leads to the bodily domination and control exercised by metropolitan imperial power. *Colonialism*, Said explains "which is almost always a consequence of imperialism, is the implanting of settlements on distant territory" (*Culture and Imperialism* 9). I find it useful to transfer this "implanting" to the region of the body since such transference would express the physical force with which colonization imprints itself on the body. This is the process that I aim to explicate by expanding on the construction of Cypriot masculinity earlier in this chapter. Yet, as I endeavour to demonstrate by focusing on dance, the process of individual corporeal colonizing takes some interesting turns.

Chapter Organization

I frame this study (chapters 1 and 5) with my experience as a "Greek Cypriot," a national identity construct that has always confounded me in both personal but also philological endeavours, complicating my subject position and invoking various anxieties. Chapter 2 follows two imperial male subjects, the French novelist Gustave Flaubert and the American journalist George William Curtis, as they journey to Upper Egypt to experience the performances of the famous dancer and courtesan Kuchuk Hanem. In a "reading" of Kuchuk's choreographies, I pose that her dancing conjured a sense of nostalgia and sexual homelessness for the imperial male.

In chapter 3, male performers of the Middle East perform against a backdrop of imperial politics. With their effeminate dress, makeup, and ornaments, male dancers exacerbated imperial anxiety felt over the male dancing body of the Orient. Ultimately, the vision of the East became crystallized in the image of the female, sexually aggressive dancer—the alternative would have implied an indulgence in sodomy.

In chapter 4 I focus on various representations of Salomé as native dancer and as decadent construct. Examining Salomé's dance (or absence thereof) in Oscar Wilde's play, I argue that Wilde fantasizes a body engaged in a dance that extends the boundaries of masculine and feminine behaviour. Through her kinesthetic excess, Salomé signals that Middle Eastern dance does not guarantee the purity of a distinct gendered or national space.

In chapter 5 I attempt some exploration of Greece's equivocal share in the legacy of Oriental dance since, although the Greek element in Oriental dance communities, especially in North America, is often strong, the intricate ways in which contemporary Greece relates to and shares in this art form remain largely unexplored. Indeed, there is a great deal to learn from the contemporary politics of "Eastern" dance in Greece since these politics host debates closely connected with Orientalism and Western imperialism. Represented as colonized space, the Greek dancing body, male and female, has measured itself and fashioned its gestures against a Eurocentric world. Having grown up in the Greek culture of

36

*Introducing
Colonial and
Postcolonial
Dialectics
on the
Subject
of Dance*

Cyprus, I share the definitions that yield constant tensions, restricting the body while promising it forms of agency.

The conclusion (chapter 6) is somewhat deceptive. Although I conclude my thoughts on various issues and attempt to tie them together, I also take advantage of the space of this chapter to discuss issues that are important to this work but are not merely conclusions. My discussion of jewellery and photographs, especially, provides further points of origin for investigation into these issues.

Despite the various mandates that I obey in this project and the variety of moods that determine the texture of the work, I consider my performance throughout mostly disciplined and well-behaved. I cite sources, comment on other critics, apply theory to my text, and I make the effort to accomplish my task with as much scholarly decency as I can assume. However, finishing the conclusion left me with the anxious notion that first, my demonstration materializes in an entirely textual production and, second, my text is marked by various inadequacies, as texts often are. Yet what troubled me the most was the need to disguise or gloss over my cathexis in the material I am dealing with. In a wish to harness the energy that emanated from this frustration, I proceeded to include an epilogue that sets out to contest textual boundaries in passages where authorial discipline and "good behaviour" are not priorities. Thus, the epilogue resists formal discussions and theories of dance and wants to become, instead, an embodied exercise in memory building. It choreographs a radical historiography and takes on political challenges *in dance*.

2 / Dismissal Veiling Desire
Kuchuk Hanem and Imperial Masculinity

But song and dance, by the very fact that they propel and animate, that is, exteriorize, have the virtues of a psychodrama played out in a closed environment. They are the equivalent of an imaginary escape from the rigid limits of the confinement, distended as long as the feast lasts.

Malek Alloula, *The Colonial Harem*

For Nerval and Flaubert, such female figures as Cleopatra, Salomé, and Isis have a special significance; and it was by no means accidental that in their work on the Orient, as well as in their visits to it, they pre-eminently valorized and enhanced female types of this legendary, richly suggestive, and associative sort.

Edward Said, *Orientalism*

M any of the travellers who left the Christian West to venture to the "heathenish" Orient in the late eighteenth and nineteenth centuries encountered a native body that they depicted as indolent, languid, and hopelessly devoid of the capitalist work ethic—an ethic that was imperative to the colonialist economy. In marked contrast, when engaged in dance, this native body transformed into a unique and ambiguous sign that provoked imperial anxiety. Indeed, few images imposed such a formidable confrontation with gender, race, and sexuality. Travellers persistently sought encounters with the dancers of the Middle East. In 1873, Charles Leland stated confidently that "the great desire of gentle-

 Notes to chapter 2 are on page 206.

38

*Dismissal
Veiling
Desire:
Kuchuk
Hanem and
Imperial
Masculinity*

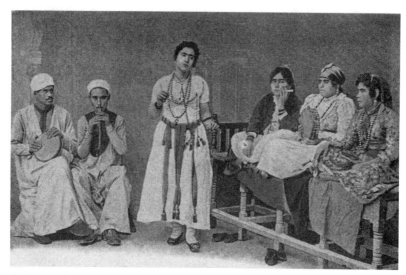

A photograph of a ghawazee dancer performing. Musicians are on her right side and seated singers on her left. It was photographed by Bonfils in the 1870s and is part of a collection of famous and much-reproduced photos taken at the same photo shoot. It was erroneously identified on the postcard as "Bedouin Dancers." (Caption by Elizabeth Artemis Mourat. Photo courtesy of University of Pennsylvania Museum, negative T2-975.)

men who come to Egypt is the dancing-girl. If it were put to the vote, most of them would prefer her to the Pyramids, if not to the Nile. Even the moral and pious, the oldest and coldest, cannot forego this bit of temptation" (130). Often these gentlemen's quest had a feverish pitch (Flaubert looked for dancers persistently), yet, paradoxically, they remained possessed by anxieties engendered by a dancer's perceived potency. Afterwards, these encounters with the Egyptian ghawazee and khawals, the Algerian ouled nayl, the Turkish çengi, among others, became a prominent feature in well-known journals, memoirs, poetry, and prose. This chapter is concerned with the cultural implications of Eastern dance for imperial male body politics. Mainly I am motivated by questions raised by the travellers' quite complex responses to the so-called Oriental body-in-motion. The sensational images evoked by Middle Eastern dancers loomed large in the Western imaginary, yet so did the ambivalent feelings for these performers. This ambivalence seems to derive from a profound need to be implicated in the aberrant spectacle so as to denounce it afterwards, in a cyclical process where disavowal succeeds desire.

The trajectory of this chapter will encompass these complex and important issues in the history of viewing Middle Eastern dance as it came, by invitation, to haunt Western ethics and disrupt cultural norms in the realm of the White West. For European travellers, the bodies of the East with their performances of excessive movement conjured images of sexual excess. This excess came to symbolize defiance and subversion despite all the efforts invested in domesticating or interpreting the dancing body in order to tame it. Although this untameable excess constitutes a behaviour that confirms Otherness and is, therefore, indispensable in the colonial encounter, it also becomes a phantasm threatening to displace the European body's sovereignty and replace it with a sexual homelessness and nostalgia, a condition that is, in turn, also indispensable. Therefore, the Western subject attempts to either "appease" the intransigent dancing body of the "Orient" by explicating it in terms of familiar markers of reference, such as Classical tradition and the Bible, or subdue it by conquering it sexually. Both approaches are attempts to exorcise the fears and anxieties generated by the "unorthodox" kinesthetics that characterize the dance of the ghawazee.

My main focus will be on the travel narratives of two eminent personalities from the West and their encounter with Kuchuk Hanem, the famous dancer and courtesan who deserves special attention in light of the issues I have outlined here.[1] Her "meeting" with Gustave Flaubert and George W. Curtis has figured in many discussions and has often been mobilized for its potential to sensationalize an interaction that has marked profoundly the East/West dynamic. However, my fascination with Kuchuk Hanem, and her admittedly fictional but nevertheless overpowering effect on me as reader, academic researcher, and dancer, has yielded the imperative to probe deeper into her association with these two men. Kuchuk's compelling persona and choreographic attraction often turn my investigation into a quest of sorts. I have felt that her body, as it emerges through narrative construction, should be capable of instituting a discourse whose possibility and potential have been disregarded. In other words, the lack of adequate theorizing of her effectual corporeality and her art has left unexplored the rich and varied implications that her fabricated presence and choreography can have on theories of dance and postcoloniality.

Performing Sex, Race, and Nostalgia

It is the evening of Wednesday, 6 March 1850. In Essna, in Upper Egypt, Kuchuk Hanem is giving a private performance for her French guests, the travelling companions Gustave Flaubert and Maxime du Camp and

40

*Dismissal
Veiling
Desire:
Kuchuk
Hanem and
Imperial
Masculinity*

their servant Joseph. The room is lit by three wicks burning in oil-filled glasses that hang on the wall in tin sconces. There is plenty of liquor, dark eyes, the clanking of coin necklaces, and European men overwhelmed by surges of physical desire. Kuchuk's companions in dance are Bambeh and Safia Zugairah and they are accompanied by musicians playing the rebab—that Lane describes as "a curious kind of viol" (370)—and darabukehs (drums). "They all sang," records an enchanted Flaubert, "the darabukehs throbbed, and the monotonous rebecs furnished a soft but shrill bass; it was like a rather gay song of mourning" (Steegmuller, *Flaubert in Egypt* 117). Flaubert has already established, earlier on the same day, that Kuchuk's dance is "brutal." In his travel notes he records her steps, evoking in the process the sexual intensity of the moment by depicting particular details:

> She squeezes her bare breasts together with her jacket. She puts on a girdle fashioned from a brown shawl with gold stripes, with three tassels hanging on ribbons. She rises first on one foot, then on the other—marvellous movement: when one foot is on the ground, the other moves up and across in front of the shin-bone—the whole thing with a light bound. I have seen this dance on old Greek vases. (*Flaubert in Egypt* 115)

This is an oneiric night for the aspiring twenty-seven-year-old Frenchman: a staged private performance for his blue eyes only, complete with musicians and a troupe of dancers who perform antiquity and Oriental sensuality for him. Between shows he has the opportunity to relish sexual intimacies with Kuchuk and her dancers. In a letter to his friend Louis Bouilhet, he tenderly refers to these moments as "intermissions for fucking" (*Letters* 116). He indulges in the occasion with devout application, as if blessed with a rare blend of mysticism, passion, tenderness, Oriental art, and most importantly, sexual intercourse with the dancer. It should not be too surprising, then, that the experience remains unique, one of the most unforgettable and celebrated in Flaubert's travels.

Many commentators, critics, and scholars have paused at this meeting, drawing some interesting and useful conclusions. A few of the passages that focus on this evening of entertainment at Kuchuk's house provide content as well as some useful information regarding both Flaubert and Kuchuk. Moreover, through these references I mean to challenge the lack of attention with which Kuchuk's dancing is most often treated. Generally, the proposition is that her dancing is an already established signifier: even if the reader has somehow not fixed the signifier for himself, any recourse to the ubiquitous Orientalist fantasies about harems and eloquent swaying would be sufficient to supply the missing signifieds. With this axiom in mind, the night of entertainment at Kuchuk's house is most often examined with ethnographic interest or seen as reiteration of stereotypical qualities. My intention is to displace such fixed and exclusive notions of Kuchuk's dancing, confident that her choreographies suggest a multivalent and dynamic terrain that calls for detailed consideration and examination.

An examination of five critics reveals fairly typical tropes in discussion. Michalis Tsianikas for example, discusses Flaubert's taste for prostitutes and his predilection for paid sexual intercourse. Prostitution, Tsianikas points out, involves a kind of love whose poetic possibility excites Flaubert and offers him an immediate aesthetic and a poetic exuberance. Kuchuk's display and marketing of her erotic charms endows her with a "masculine" quality and, apparently, Flaubert has always found masculine women irresistible (Tsianikas 65). For Kuchuk, however, it seems that this "masculine" quality is a corollary of her status. According to Fatima Mernissi, a woman in Islamic society is not considered biologically inferior to a man (as Flaubert and Curtis believed), and is perceived, instead, as a powerful and dangerous being. Indeed, Kuchuk transgresses laws as she exists and operates outside established social and sexual institutions (such as polygamy, sexual segregation, and legal subordination in the family structure) which have served male strategies intended to contain female power (19).[2] Wendy Buonaventura dwells on Flaubert's melancholy attachment to Kuchuk and her lasting impression on him. Buonaventura suggests that Flaubert purposely cultivated the melancholy aspect of his amorousness in order to extract to the full the bittersweet nature of an encounter with a courtesan (76-77). Judith Tucker relies on the same travel narrative to reach some conclusions about Kuchuk's skills and talents, as well as her economic and social status in relation to the repercussions of her banishment from Cairo as a result of the 1834 edict. Tucker finds that on her evening with Flaubert, Kuchuk "danced, played, and sang with a grace and skill bespeaking a past with the *awâlim*" (152), the learned female performers. In his seminal work *Orientalism*, Edward Said discusses the same event as a paradigm that exemplifies the thesis of his book:

> [Flaubert] was foreign, comparatively wealthy, male, and these were historical facts of domination that allowed him not only to posses Kuchuk Hanem physically but to speak for her and tell his readers in what way she was "typically Oriental." My argument is that Flaubert's situation of

42

Dismissal
Veiling
Desire:
Kuchuk
Hanem and
Imperial
Masculinity

strength in relation to Kuchuk Hanem was not an isolated instance. It fairly stands for the pattern of relative strength between East and West, and the discourse about the Orient that it enabled. (6)

Said makes the rather predictable observation that Kuchuk is "the prototype of Flaubert's Salambô and Salomé, as well as of all the versions of carnal female temptation to which his Saint Anthony is subject" (187). While these influences are useful to note (and I will discuss them in some detail in chapter 4), critics do not seem to encourage what I find to be a necessary scope: radical and in-depth consideration of Kuchuk's choreographies and the intricacies of their influence that marked the dynamic of the encounter.

Travelling up the Nile to Upper Egypt earlier the same year, January of 1850, was George William Curtis, an American "essayist, author, orator, and publicist" (Monty 126). Like Flaubert, he sought Kuchuk Hanem and devotes to her and her talents two entire chapters in *Nile Notes of a Howadji*, the travelogue that details his travels. He refers to her in a variety of mixed metaphors and appellations, all of which are important indicators of his own subject position in relation to her gender and racial identification as well as her art. His favourite reference is to Terpsichore, the muse of dance in Grecian mythology. Chapter 20 in *Nile Notes* is a detailed account of the evening of entertainment at Kuchuk Hanem's house, or "bower" as he calls it, and he entitles the entire chapter after the muse since he sees the Egyptian dancer as the metempsychosis of Terpsichore.

Unlike Flaubert, however, Curtis feigns a certain coyness at those moments when the intimation of sexual intensity is too powerful to ignore. Such a moment is the detailed description of Kuchuk's dress, for example, when his gaze traverses the dancer's body, feigning to depict details of dress but relaying a concealed undercurrent of sexual voyeurism in the act. Another such oxymoronic moment occurs when Xenobi hands him the nargileh, an elaborate Eastern smoking apparatus (also known as a *hookah*). She is one of the young members of Kuchuk's ensemble and for Curtis she is "a very dove of a Ghazeeyah, a quiet child, the last born of Terpsichore" (135). Her gesture signifies for him "an electric chain of communication" (135), as the nargileh's "serpentine sinuosity flowed through her fingers, as if the golden gayety of her costume were gliding from her alive" (135). Throughout his account he carefully maintains an ambivalent stance as he deploys his virtue against the temptations of the erotically excessive Orient embodied by the ghawazee. This ambivalence becomes manifest in that he reads the signs and registers the sensuality, yet he consciously masks his reading by deploying the guise of the erudite Westerner whose learning affords him an almost ascetic and, certainly, detached stance. His *Nile Notes*, therefore, are keen to portray a traveller with a certain informed innocence, the oxymoron suggesting Mary Louise Pratt's "seeing-man," a term that Curtis qualifies for. Pratt coins this "admittedly unfriendly label" (7) to describe a particular kind of imperial man on tour. The "seeing-man" denotes a subject who, in his travel and exploration, employs strategies of innocence while also asserting imperial hegemony. Pratt believes "these strategies of innocence are constituted in relation to older imperial rhetorics of conquest associated with the absolutist era" (7). Curtis is undoubtedly a modern embodiment of the observant and curious, indefatigable, bourgeois subject whose task is to record what he sees in order to titillate, educate, and ultimately reassert the superiority of his own ideology to his own people: white, bourgeois, American readers.

Interestingly, in Middle Eastern dance research and also in critical scholarship on travel writing, Flaubert's meeting with Kuchuk receives more attention than Curtis's account. Perhaps the unabashed explicitness of Flaubert's account is too provocative to resist. Curtis's description of her dancing is, however, a great deal more detailed, with an apparent attempt at precision. I quote at length:

> Kuchuk Arnem [sic] rose and loosened her shawl girdle in such wise, that I feared she was about to shed the frivolity of dress, as Venus shed the sea foam, and stood opposite the divan, holding her brass castanets.... [She] stood motionless, while this din deepened around her.... The sharp surges of sound swept around the room, dashing in regular measure against her movelessness, until suddenly the whole surface of her frame quivered in measure with the music. Her hands were raised, clapping the castanets, and she slowly turned upon herself, her right leg the pivot, marvellously convulsing all the muscles of her body. When she completed the circuit of the spot on which she stood, she advanced slowly, all the muscles jerking in time to the music, and in solid, substantial spasms. It was a curious and wonderful gymnastic. There was no graceful dancing—once only there was the movement of dancing, when she advanced, throwing one leg before the other as gipsies dance. But the rest was most voluptuous motion—not the lithe wooing of languid passion, but the soul of passion starting through every sense, and quivering in every limb. It was the very intensity of motion, concentrated and constant. The music still swelled savagely, in maddened monotony of measure. Hecate and the old hus-

44

*Dismissal
Veiling
Desire:
Kuchuk
Hanem and
Imperial
Masculinity*

band, fascinated with the Ghazeeyah's fire, threw their hands and arms excitedly about their instruments, and an occasional cry of enthusiasm and satisfaction burst from their lips. Suddenly stooping, still muscularly moving, Kushuk [*sic*] fell upon her knees, and writhed, with body, arms, and head upon the floor, still in measure—still clanking the castanets, and arose in the same manner. It was profoundly dramatic. The scenery of the dance was like that of a characteristic song. It was a lyric of love, which words cannot tell—profound, oriental, intense, and terrible. Still she retreated, until the constantly down-slipping shawl seemed only just clinging to her hips, and making the same circuit upon herself, she sat down, and after this violent and extravagant exertion she was marbly cold. (140-42)[3]

This passage provides enough detail about Kuchuk's dancing to enable some speculation on choreographies of the ghawazee in the mid-nineteenth century. In fact, some of the moves, as relayed through Curtis's interpretation, appear to be somewhat reminiscent of popular contemporary Oriental dance moves, such as the shimmy, suggested by the quivering frame, and the slow turn with muscular convulsions while the body balances on one leg.[4] Moreover, the complete body control of the dancer is perceptible even in Curtis's translation and so is the spiritual and ecstatic element of the dance. These qualities become manifest in the apparent divorce of the body from its material surroundings and a complete identification with what is driving it. Even when physical space is not restricted, expression relies mainly on movement of the arms, head, and torso while steps are small and legs are used to assist the performance but not to cover physical space. All of these movements that are quite intense in proportion to their physical compass are characteristic of Oriental dance in its contemporary interpretations. Both Berger (11) and Monty (134) have also suggested similar readings of this scene, applying it to modern renditions of the dance.[5] Kuchuk's motionlessness, especially, is a powerful kinesthetic moment that enhances her expression just as strongly as her quivering. In the process of exoticization, which Curtis follows meticulously, he seems to suggest that there is a certain spirit imbuing the dancer's body slowly and steadily. Furthermore, the enthusiasm of the dance inspires those present and dominates the atmosphere. Admittedly, Curtis's choice of diction here is quite engaging, with his reference to the dance as "scenery" and song, thus making all kinds of other cross-references and images possible. He is certainly comfortable in his domain of the privileged Western viewer. Such phrases as "profound, intense, terrible," distance him even further, the gesture increasing his safety and reducing his readers' anxiety during this sensitive moment when the Empire is undergoing various tests while witnessing this spectacle. A rather telling moment demonstrating his ease as a distinguished voyeur is his reference to the shawl girdle, the adorning item described as a prologue to Kuchuk's dancing. She loosens it in a gesture that supposedly incites fear in Curtis, as it threatens to expose before his chaste gaze the shocking nudity of an Eastern body. This is clearly a moment when the dance is made into a spectacle through the common trope of imminent nudity, an odd prospect considering that Kuchuk was dressed underneath the shawl. Curtis's purpose, however, is to titillate the (male) reader by staging the spectacle for his readers in a sexually threatening—in other words enticing—manner but then rescuing the reader just at the last moment.

Yet, how far can one go with these interpretations of Kuchuk's dance? Edward Said's comments about her in *Orientalism* fall within the larger schema of his arguments, and would, therefore, be subject to the various criticisms that have been levelled against this work. Aijaz Ahmad, for example, in his elaborate critique of Said, objects to the sweeping temporal and geographical reach of the book. He argues that Said's ambition in *Orientalism* gets out of control as Said expands the Orient geographically through the book until it finally reaches from Morocco to the Far East. Also, Said's premise is that since the age of Classical Athens (identified as the "West") the Orient has been under construction by the West and this pattern has not seen significant changes over the last twenty-five centuries. These are only two of the problems that Ahmad locates and protests against, vehemently at times, and which make him contend that *Orientalism* is "a deeply flawed book" (161).[6] In terms of Ahmad's objections, Kuchuk is merely a monolithic representation of the available woman of the East, "peculiarly Oriental in her luxuriant and seemingly unbounded sexuality" (187), deprived of volition or agency. Concerning Middle Eastern dance, Said avoids the challenge of a closer focus on Kuchuk's movement, relying instead on a formulaic treatment of the activity in colonial discourse; the East, totally objectified, performs for the West. Kuchuk is not an individual or even an artist but a figure as vague and far-reaching geographically and temporally as the Orient in Said's work.

Said avoids the challenge also because dance often inhibits with its evanescence.[7] Unlike the written word, a dance move is executed literally and figuratively. It transpires just at the moment the body gives it life. Observing its motion, the gaze struggles to fix and secure those rapid

Dismissal
Veiling
Desire:
Kuchuk
Hanem and
Imperial
Masculinity

frames of movement that form only to vanish upon appearance. Indeed, the dancing body eludes capture in any material terms, hence the reluctance of critics such as Said, Tucker, Tsianikas, and even Buonaventura to discuss the movement itself. Indeed, it feels much safer to discuss a written memoir or a travelogue rather than a choreographed moment that reaches us through the European viewer's often poor translation. Despite such weaknesses, it is the native dancing body that often becomes the fetishized sign of eroticism, passion, unbridled sexuality, or even a symbol of savagery and brutality. Perhaps we need to focus on these attributes of dance as the object of celebration and not anxiety—although, in a Western context where validity is guaranteed only by inscription, we may have lost the means to register and consume these experiences imaginatively. Nevertheless, we should dare to urge the dance to speak even from the confines of a journalistic interpretation. What are the implications of Kuchuk's choreographies, as bequeathed to us by Flaubert and George W. Curtis, on colonial discourse and theories of dance? In other words, can we not focus on the movement itself in order to draw some conclusions about Europe's perception of Middle Eastern dance in the context of colonialism? As it vanishes, does dance leave signs on the imperial body—signs that may disclose important narratives about this body's contact with the Middle Eastern dancing body?

Kuchuk's Dance and Flaubert's Performance

While on his Oriental tour, almost concurrently with Curtis, Flaubert claims to desire to speak the Orient differently from his literary predecessors (Tsianikas 132). Thus, he breaks with the Romantic tradition that venerated remnants of the revered civilizations of Classical Greece, Rome, and, to a certain extent, Ancient Egypt. He claims indifference to erudition and culture and seeks, instead, Egypt's dancers who embody what the Empire finds reprehensible and whose promise includes a raw and intense sexual fulfillment. In fact, he makes this embodiment the object of his study, indulging his obsession with the Eastern body and defying even further the noble concerns of his predecessors. Kuchuk offers him the perfect opportunity for Oriental spectacle as well as sexual fulfillment, alluring him with the eroticism that Flaubert seems to find implicit in her dance. In her movement he sees reified a sexual invitation evoking the desire to possess the body whose ontological existence and performance find their meaning only in the evocation of his pleasure.

Furthermore, her dance is a sensuous celebration of the body that contrasts strikingly with the disciplined European bodies that he knows, male and female. As Flaubert knew it, the European female body, perceived as the repository of sexuality, is especially disciplined by being forced into a set, restrictive form that repudiates its natural shape. Thus, in a discourse that construes the body as the intransigent agent of sexual deviance, its unruliness is contained in stays often fitted with metal straps. This treatment aims at reshaping it into a form whose sadistic confinement and artificial definition inform the dominant aesthetic. Writing to his uncle, Monsieur Parain, from Constantinople (only a few months after his Egyptian tour), Flaubert laments the changes in Eastern dress that he fears are imminent.[8] Describing the veiled women on the streets of Constantinople in all the terms familiar from European colonial discourse, Flaubert exclaims: "To think—oh misery!—that in ten years they will be in hat and corset, imitating their husbands who already dress like Europeans, in shoes and overcoats!" (Steegmuller, *Flaubert and Madame Bovary* 200). In the dancing that Flaubert experiences in Kuchuk's house, the dancers' motions seem to contradict the European body's socially defined contour and there seems to be a greater acceptance of the body's natural form. His excitement over Kuchuk's performance of "The Bee" is intricately connected to these body politics. This is a "mythical dance" whose name alone survives, as Flaubert informs us, and whose excitement is in the nudity it involves. "Kuchuk shed her clothing as she danced" (*Flaubert in Egypt* 117) and, as Marjorie Garber posits, "a curious feature of this dance is its aura of taboo: the musicians and other necessary members of the dancer's entourage are themselves veiled or blindfolded during the performance" (341). I believe, however, that Flaubert's claim to be subjugated by this particular performance stems largely not so much from the taboo but from the ecphrasis (the vivid and profound articulation) realized by the dancing body: it simultaneously becomes the incarnation of his longing as well as a visionary disclosure of his own captured/incarcerated body.

In my effort to interpret Flaubert's responses to the contrasts he finds noteworthy between his own cultural milieu and the Orient, the parameters of art, fashion, and social behaviour come into strong play especially as they are reflected in dance. The oppressive motif of "hat and corset" that Flaubert discerns in European women's dress finds its expression in prescribed feminine behaviour and gesture. In artistic terms this motif emerges in ballet dance performance that, in some ways, emulates

Dismissal
Veiling
Desire:
Kuchuk
Hanem and
Imperial
Masculinity

acceptable femininity and propriety. Therefore, to delineate the contrast between European ballerinas and Middle Eastern dancers is quite necessary for a more complete understanding of Flaubert's reaction to Kuchuk. In ballet the female dancer attempts to become almost invisible, rising en pointe and stretching into the vertical, whereas a Middle Eastern dancer emphasizes a horizontal, grounded dimension that engages an entirely different set of signifiers. In his article that commemorates the passing of Tahia Carioca, one of Egypt's most famous dancers of the twentieth century, Edward Said delineates the contrasts between these two dance forms:

> Belly dancing in many ways is the opposite of ballet, its Western equivalent as an art form. Ballet is all about elevation, lightness, the defiance of the body's weight. Eastern dancing as Tahia practiced it shows the dancer planting herself more and more solidly in the earth, digging into it almost, scarcely moving, certainly never expressing anything like the nimble semblance of weightlessness that a great ballet dancer, male or female, tries to convey. ("Farewell to Tahia" 230)

While Said here seems concerned mainly with belly dance as it developed for a cabaret setting, his comments encompass a wider aesthetic of Eastern dance versus ballet. They are, therefore, quite useful in this context since this contrasting negotiation of space and meaning is one of the attractions that draw Flaubert to Middle Eastern dance, leaving him evidently indifferent to ballet.

Of course, the iconoclastic attitude Flaubert adopted while on tour is not as radical as he likes to believe since his sensibility has been shaped by the same bourgeois narratives that became the foundation of an imperialist European system. The classics and the Bible, as well as a Romantic construct of Egypt and its monumental grandeur, have marked him as well. For example, while on his Oriental tour, he contemplates Byron intensely, especially at Abydos. This cognitive tribute to the Romantic English poet reveals a sensitive attachment to a certain poetic tradition, perhaps even a certain anxious longing to form part of that tradition. It also reveals a certain camaraderie that attaches itself to an exotic place, the apex of this love triangle that now becomes mapped as a point of reference for a Western literary male figure. Echoing Byron's need for a tour, Flaubert travels to Egypt motivated by curiosity and a need to escape from social confines and experience the spectacle of the East. Rana Kabbani has commented on the pre-existence of this Eastern vision in his mind's eye long before he embarked on his tour:

When he finally arrived in Egypt in 1849, he could write that its atmosphere had the nature of a "retrouvaille." The landscape had already been imprinted in his imagination, culled from the Bible and from Oriental accounts and paintings.... The real voyage for Flaubert served mainly to authenticate the imaginary one. When he arrived in the Orient, he saw an East he had transported with him; one that he would transport back, in piecemeal, in the form of extravagant objects. (71-72)

When he first visits Kuchuk's house in eager anticipation, he celebrates the occasion by depicting her in images rather common in travel-journal orthodoxy. She emerges in a literal sense from her bath and in a figurative sense like Aphrodite: "she had just come from the bath, her firm breasts had a fresh smell, something like that of sweetened turpentine; she began by perfuming her hands with rose water" (Steegmuller, *Flaubert in Egypt* 114). She has the aura of a Mother Earth figure, mystical and imposing. His description is a ritualistic recreation of Kuchuk and he seems to relish the process as if it's an erotic substitute. She is a heavenly sphere silhouetted against the sun, an earth suspended in a bright Oriental sky. She is "on the stairs, opposite us, surrounded by light and standing against the background of the blue sky." Soon, the landscape of her body emerges in a description as monumental as the land of Egypt itself:

> When she bends, her flesh ripples into bronze ridges. Her eyes are dark and enormous. Her eyebrows black, her nostrils open and wide; heavy shoulders, full, apple-shaped breasts.... Her black hair, wavy, unruly, pulled straight back on each side form a center parting beginning at the forehead; small braids joined together at the nape of her neck. She has one upper incisor, right, which is beginning to go bad. For a bracelet she has two bands of gold, twisted together and interlaced, around one wrist. Triple necklace of large hollow gold beads. Earrings: gold disks, slightly convex, circumference decorated with gold granules. (*Flaubert in Egypt* 114-15)

Juxtaposing adjectives, Flaubert seems anxious to force a certain metaphysical potential he perceives in Kuchuk. At once she is mortal and divine and as appealing as the Orient itself: dark and enormous, black, open, wide, and unruly. But she is also mortal and Flaubert can relish his mystic vision only through an unrelenting evocation of mortality. The reference to the bad tooth, in characteristic Flaubertian precision, forces temporality upon this formidable woman, thus reducing her awesome appearance through an unkind reference to a marker of decay and mutability that will eventually consume her.[9] At the same time, however, he wants her to be continuing an ancient tradition. Keen on acting as the

*Dismissal
Veiling
Desire:
Kuchuk
Hanem and
Imperial
Masculinity*

European scholar in possession of the gaze (*her* dark eyes are not given vision), he attempts to record and confine her linguistically. Yet even at this moment, Flaubert is revealing his own weakness and abjection since his observations gesture towards limitations (mutability, decay) from which the writer himself is far from being exempt.

In Flaubert's panorama, Kuchuk Hanem's body comes to replace the ancient monuments which he insists leave him indifferent. Nevertheless, during the tour he studies Greek and reads Homer every day (*Letters* 114). Moreover, Kuchuk's dancing is familiar to him from "old Greek vases" (Steegmuller, *Flaubert in Egypt* 115), a comment illustrative of a long tradition he recognizes in her dance, yet also characteristic of colonial discourse. As Said has observed about a Western person's visit to the Orient,

> one tends to stop judging things either as completely novel or as completely well known; a new median category emerges, a category that allows one to see new things, things seen for the first time, as versions of a previously known thing. In essence such a category is not so much a way of receiving new information as it is a method of controlling what seems to be a threat to some established view of things. (*Orientalism* 58-59)

In Flaubert's remark, representations on the vases of Greek antiquity and the dancer in front of him are conflated, emphasizing the continuity of the dance through the ages and cultures. Even though Said is not referring specifically to Flaubert, his description resonates with what Flaubert needs to control: his established view of the ancient past, and more specifically, the connections between Greece and Egypt. They are both the same Orient whose culture survives unaltered through time. In a certain sense, Flaubert's comment could also attest to his iconoclastic attitude towards the literary legacy of Europe. Specifically, Greece is not the classical land that gave birth to Western refinement but a land of unruly potential with women who engage in orgiastic Bacchic rituals depicted on Attic vases. In any case, not only are Greece and Egypt conflated into one Orient but also the ancient past is still alive and dancing, and for him, with his elite education and with these ancient civilizations as cultural background, Kuchuk's performance has the atmosphere of a "retrouvaille." I see, therefore, an implicit attempt to break with tradition except that this attempt is informed by tradition itself. Flaubert's rendition of the experience thwarts his own scope.

Following the wild party, Flaubert lies with Kuchuk to practise the only choreography he is adept at. As he dozes off, with his fingers clasping her fetishized necklace, the image that flashes through his mind is biblical: Judith and Holofernes (*Flaubert in Egypt* 118. I will return to discuss the significance of this recurring image and its implications in chapter 4). Later, she sleeps and snores while he is vigilant and contemplative. In fact, the effect of her choreography and what it induced in Flaubert is manifest not only in the immediate scant depiction of her dance but afterwards when he is sharing her bed. He writes to Louis Bouilhet:

> I sucked her furiously, her body was covered with sweat, she was tired after dancing, she was cold. I covered her with my fur pelisse, and she fell asleep.... As for me, I scarcely shut my eyes. My night was one long, infinitely intense reverie. That was why I stayed. Watching that beautiful creature asleep (she snored, her head against my arm ...), I thought of my nights in Paris brothels ... and I thought of her, of her dance, of her voice as she sang songs that were for me without meaning and even without distinguishable words. (*Letters* 117)

He "sucks furiously" as if to consume some spirit that possessed her during the dance. The spirit, however, has departed, leaving the body cold and Flaubert desiring what he will inevitably be denied. Kuchuk's art remains a signifier without a referent for Flaubert, who feels compelled to supply one himself, almost blindly. While Kuchuk is snoring he is alert and self-gazing, watching his ineffectual presence beside this woman, unable to formulate any meaning, his imperial subjectivity incapable of securing him a safe arrival at the site he yearns for. His mental processes counterbalance his kinesthetic lack. While Kuchuk's dancing body marks space and time, Flaubert's body is inert, his eyes gazing at the spectacle. When Kuchuk is asleep he is vigilant, the moment being appropriate for him to engage in some kind of mental activity that will parallel Kuchuk's dance. This activity involves an almost conscious attempt to exoticize Kuchuk and I would like to underscore the imperative of this process as it allows Flaubert to mark gender, racial, and cultural difference. Or, as Marta Savigliano would put it, exoticism creates the abstract, unfulfillable desire to attain completeness in the colonized while extracting his or her passion.[10] This desire is what overwhelms not only the French writer's letter to his male friend but also Curtis's description as well. Such yearning for completeness then, becomes the canonical feeling in narratives by male travellers.

In his notes, but not in the letter, Flaubert articulates with unexpected directness and clarity one of the motivating thoughts that generate this mixture of yearning and anxiety: "How flattering it would be to

Dismissal
Veiling
Desire:
Kuchuk
Hanem and
Imperial
Masculinity

one's pride if at the moment of leaving you were sure that you left a memory behind, that she would think of you more than of the others who
have been there, that you would remain in her heart!" (Steegmuller,
Flaubert in Egypt 119).

Morroe Berger distills the histrionics of Flaubert's lament in a sentence whose reductionism and unenlightened simplicity are disturbing:
"This is the vain dream of the romantic young artist: to leave an impression upon the whore" (33). To this day dancers suffer from similar imperialist and misogynist onslaughts intended to denigrate them to specific
and familiar abject roles. Flaubert's scenario with Kuchuk is, of course, a
great deal more complex. Evidently, his priority is to endeavour that kind
of intercourse with the Orient that will render his name inexhaustible.
Flaubert is eager to construct this encounter with Kuchuk as a sacred
ritual from which he can emerge transformed and immortal. He enjoys
the privilege of having the East perform before his gaze but he also
acknowledges a certain power in the dancer that subdues him, turning
him into an overpowered subjectivity. His European learning turns against
him as it helps to generate the barely conscious realization that the East
was there long before he arrived, stretching from classical antiquity to the
tombs of the Pharaohs and the Sphinx. Also, the dance itself is evidence
of a long tradition of female creativity and religious celebration. Indeed,
the Orient does not need Flaubert as much as he needs it, hence Flaubert's
almost desperate attempt to unite with the Orient as it is condensed in
this dancer's body. On her body he inscribes his physical desire, insa-
tiably pouring himself inside Kuchuk as if to drown any other kind of
ecstasy she is capable of experiencing. Now, not surprisingly, he wants
his subjectivity inscribed in her heart; he wants to secure sole rights to
her passion.

It is another strange moment of ambivalence: he possesses her body
with a feeling of submission to this powerful courtesan; he is an imperial
subject yet he seeks refuge in the woman's physical and emotional domain:
it is almost an expression of hopelessness. This crisis seems directly linked
to Kuchuk's choreographies. Her movement incites his fixation in a
dynamic that lends force to Homi Bhabha's argument that the colonial
encounter cannot be contained in simple binary and mutually exclusive
oppositions. Flaubert's stereotypical concept of Kuchuk embodies mas-
tery and anxiety simultaneously as it divides him internally. She becomes
the "impossible object." In Homi Bhabha's words, the "exertions of the
'official knowledges of colonialism ... are imbricated at the point of their

production of meaning and power with the fantasy that dramatizes the impossible desire for a pure, undifferentiated origin" (81). Flaubert's night with Kuchuk may also be observed as an enactment of what Bhabha describes in his discussion on the stereotype and colonialist discourse as a "scene of fetishism." As he enters that complicated economy of "love" during those very intimate moments, Flaubert becomes an actor in "the scene of the reactivation and repetition of primal fantasy—the subject's desire for a pure origin that is always threatened by its division, for the subject must be gendered to be engendered, to be spoken" (75). What Bhabha identifies as "pure origin" haunts Flaubert's dialogism, at that vulnerable moment when he seeks to be divided in order to discover wholeness.

It would seem that Egypt's dancers could offer Flaubert something exquisite that he could not find in Parisian prostitutes. Possessing the exotic dancer's body enhances the meaning of carnal conquest, as well as imperial conquest by extension, and offers pleasurable fulfillment as well as an abode of sorts. Put in the words of Malek Alloula, Kuchuk's song and dances can be "the equivalent of an imaginary escape from the rigid limits of confinement distended as long as the feast lasts" (86). Along with the recognition that this dance is a surviving art form with an ancient history (by "recognition" I am thinking of *anagnorisis* from ancient Greek drama, a sudden awareness that overwhelms the consciousness), comes the understanding that it extends beyond his temporal constraints as a Western viewer.

Furthermore, the nature of the dance itself, its suppleness, and the ritualistic quality of the performance appear to the spectator to challenge physical restrictions, its motion stretching the body's potential for expression. In fact, contemporary discussions of the tradition of this dance insist that the dancing body is endowed with a certain sanctity. Wendy Buonaventura, for example, believes that "the trance, or ecstatic element, was crucial, for it released an energy in the body which helped the dancer enter into another realm of experience and unite with the deity, whose power was thus transferred to her" (31). Similarly, in Dionysian or primitive Mother Earth rituals, ecstasy achieved through the dance signified spiritual union with the goddess or god, the *enthousiasmos* that Lillian Lawler discusses as ecstatic union with the divine, "the state of having the god within one" ("Terpsichore" 27). This notion of ecstatic union is a popular conviction that has greatly influenced modern interpretations of Middle Eastern dance.

*Dismissal
Veiling
Desire:
Kuchuk
Hanem and
Imperial
Masculinity*

Yet I cannot help but wonder how much of this discourse Kuchuk would be aware of. How did she feel the dance in her body? Did she possess that spiritual dimension of dance that many women today lay claim to? These questions (although unanswerable) might be helpful in assessing Flaubert's role in his meeting with Kuchuk. If he saw the dance on Greek vases, then he may have been conscious of meanings associated with spirituality, ecstasy, and ritual. Perhaps even he had been on a quest for such meanings. Clearly, though, the character of the dance is made to coincide with notions of the East itself (enthralling, spiritual, sensual, primeval), so that in Flaubert's imagination the ghaziya (singular of ghawazee) and Egypt are conflated into a rather vague metaphor for Oriental exoticism. In this conflation lies the formula that I complained about earlier. However, Kuchuk's performance requires his voyeuristic gaze and her courtesan occupation allows him access to her physical body. This exchange sets up an economy in which Flaubert feels he has a control that fascinates him with its totality. What he seems to perceive is that having sexual access to the body whose serpentine movements and formidable agility achieve a divine ecstasy means, ultimately, possession of timeless Oriental magic. This is the fantasy. However, her dance leaves traces on his body—traces of sexual homelessness and nostalgia that ensue and overwhelm his *enthousiasmos*.

There can be little doubt that, on a practical level at least, Kuchuk's perspective must have differed greatly. Surely, her performance was an economic exchange that earned her a living. She does not wish her guests to stay overnight, since burglars who know about their visit might attempt to break in and steal her jewellery, which Judith Tucker believes to be a memento from Kuchuk's older and more prosperous times (152). Because such economies may very well have been at play, there may even have existed a certain element of auto-exoticism in her performance, an effort to offer the wealthy visiting patron the product that he expected to receive. In fact, in this context of auto-exoticization, it seems to me that Kuchuk's striking gesture of squeezing her bare breasts together and tying her jacket around them could perhaps indicate a performativity intended for consumption.

Flaubert is left suspended between his physical desire, which seeks to inscribe itself on her body, and his mental (unfulfilled) desire to occupy the space that she defines for herself. In the aftermath of his Oriental tour these limitations become salient. In a telling letter to Louise Colet he attempts a pragmatic, yet deeply troubling, analysis of his affair with Kuchuk:

As for Kuchuk Hanem, ah! Set your mind at rest, and at the same time correct your ideas about the Orient. You may be sure that she felt nothing at all: emotionally, I guarantee; and even physically, I strongly suspect. She found us very good cawadjas (seigneurs), because we left a goodly number of piastres behind, that's all…. The oriental woman is no more than a machine: she makes no distinction between one man and another. Smoking, going to the baths, painting her eyelids and drinking coffee—such is the circle of occupations within which her existence is confined. As for physical pleasure, it must be very slight, since the famous button, the seat thereof, is sliced off at an early age. What makes this woman, in a sense, so poetic, is that she relapses into the state of nature. (*Letters*, 181)

Subdued and rather dejected, the tone here may be intended as merely a gesture to appease Louise. Nevertheless, the passage seems to navigate through various sites that need to be identified and examined. Lisa Lowe finds Flaubert's description unsettling and discusses it as "paradigmatic of the intersections of and collusions between several nineteenth-century French discourses, not only of orientalism and romanticism but also of race and industrial capitalism" (76). Lowe demonstrates how, far from being a singularized or monolithic representation, Kuchuk inhabits a complex topos where a multiplicity of discourses and social relations cross. The dancer emerges in various embodiments: as an eroticized female figure posing in the tradition of orientalist iconography, sexual enchantress but also inspiring romantic muse; and as a dehumanized machine that this description makes racially inferior.

I find Lowe's analysis of the layered implications of this problematic passage to be quite astute. But it is important to point out that the falsehood, inaccuracies, and stereotypes that mark this letter seem to index a strong attempt to dismiss the experience in order to manage a sense of release. There is a tone of misogyny that becomes an unwarranted defence in his comment that the "Oriental woman" is a machine—an image obfuscated by Kuchuk's apparently poetic ability to relapse into a state of nature. Moreover, much of his frustration stems from the realization that he has not been the distinguished guest to mark Kuchuk, or indeed any ghaziya, with a lasting impression. And then, the courtesan's routine, outlined in a fashion that solicits derision, contempt, and rejection, is a decadent lifestyle which Flaubert himself enjoyed during his travels to the Orient as well as at home in Paris. He seems keen to curtail this woman's independence by outlining her dependence on habits considered frivolous in the dogma of a capitalist work ethic. Makeup seems to contest this

Dismissal
Veiling
Desire:
Kuchuk
Hanem and
Imperial
Masculinity

ethic by imposing a ritual of a purely personal and vain indulgence (see the discussion of kohl in chapter 1). He also knows that the sketch he provides is not a fair representation of her life, subject as she is to the harshness of mortality (suggested by Flaubert's description of her incisor "which is beginning to go bad") and to her material circumstances (she is anxious about her physical safety while in her own house). However, as Homi Bhabha indicates,

> Stereotyping is not the setting up of a false image which becomes the scapegoat of discriminatory practices. It is a much more ambivalent text of projection and introjection, metaphoric and metonymic strategies, displacement, overdetermination, guilt, aggressivity; the masking and splitting of "official" and phantasmatic knowledges to construct the positionalities and oppositionalities of racist discourse. (81-82)

Bhabha's complication of imperialist, racist discourse is a good way to account for Flaubert's complex discursive construct of his position. In simple terms, he assures Colet that she has no reason to feel rivalry over Kuchuk who is nothing but an "Oriental woman." For her, one man is presumably the same as the next so long as he pays for her leisure time and frivolous habits, especially adornment. This attempt to convey the "official" Oriental knowledge masks the phantasmatic construction of Kuchuk as well as of himself in relation to her. Despite its apparent simplicity, Flaubert's racist stereotype involves the complicated trope that Bhabha is suggesting, particularly the projections of desire onto Kuchuk and the displacement, which I interpret as "sexual homelessness."

Finally, in Flaubert's letter to Colet, his comment that Kuchuk received a clitoridectomy at a young age comes as a shock, since in his travel notes he refrains from commenting on this fact—if indeed it is a fact. Flaubert's obliqueness gives rise to speculation: does he refrain from mentioning it in order to enhance the effect of his sexual performance as he describes it to Louis Bouilhet, his keen receiver? Or does he want to avoid the thought that even during sexual intercourse he is denied every form of accommodation he seeks in this woman? Whatever the case might be, if what he relates here is indeed factual, Kuchuk's alleged impotence at feeling pleasure is another way in which Flaubert's fantasy of sexual fulfilment, as well as his grandiose sense of himself as provider of sexual pleasure, is frustrated and replaced instead with a fantasy of his own impotence. His final gesture in this very problematic attempt at defending his inadequacies is to connect the dancer with the "state of nature." This comment, like his previous, is also somewhat obscure. However one wishes to interpret it, the romanticized Kuchuk becomes the female savage endowed with a certain nobility because of her primitive capacity to live in her "natural" self and be in harmony with her humanity, if not sexual pleasure, through kinesthetic ecstasy. A moment when Flaubert's sexual homelessness and nostalgia for Kuchuk are strongly manifest occurs while he travels through Turkey. Here he misses her greatly and his words reveal the extent of his fixation on her and his nostalgic attachment to the dancer but also to his close friend Louis Bouilhet: "Why have I a melancholy desire to return to Egypt, to go back up the Nile and see Kuchuk Hanem? All the same, it was a rare night I spent there, and I tasted it to the full. How I missed you!" (*Letters* 131).

Curtis, on the other hand, tries to keep his interpersonal dynamics less complicated. He declares his presence in Egypt in terms of a surveying monarch, the person who mediates between Empire and the peripheral lands. Occupying such an intermediate position, this emissary suffers the obligation to observe and transcribe geographical space, interiors, and native bodies in order to re-present them to the metropolitan centre, thus fulfilling the subject's duties of loyalty to the imperial project. Throughout, Curtis seems conscious that the privilege which the gaze almost invariably confers is equivocated by the exertion of having to perform the imperial subject in the contact zone. In the space of the contact zone, Mary Louise Pratt explains, "peoples geographically and historically separated come into contact with each other and establish ongoing relations, usually involving conditions of coercion, radical inequality, and intractable conflict" (6). Using his erudite expertise, Curtis manipulates Kuchuk's dance, depicting it simultaneously as a choreographed assault on Western propriety and morals and, while assuming St. George's panoply, he fends off the evil and destruction unleashed by her native dance.[11] All the while, Curtis treats his readers to a male heterosexual voyeuristic indulgence, complete with the subtle pornographic touches of young fingers handling phallic objects such as the nargileh with its "serpentine sinuosity."

Negotiating White Subjectivity

One of the challenges, then, in examining how Flaubert's and Curtis's different travel narratives enact the imperial gaze upon the ghaziya's body, concerns the ways in which this gaze negotiates personal and imperial interests while maintaining loyalty to the Empire, and coping with the dis-

Dismissal
Veiling
Desire:
Kuchuk
Hanem and
Imperial
Masculinity

comfort of pressure that the contact zone almost invariably entails. In the words of James Duncan and Derek Gregory, "even in its most imperial gestures, by virtue of its occupation of that 'space in-between'—the space of transculturation—travel writing can also disclose an ambivalence, a sense of its own authorities and assumptions being called into question" (*Writes of Passage* 5). In an effort to cope with these challenges, sustain authority, and enhance confidence in their assumptions, Flaubert and Curtis sought recourse to the canons that formed bourgeois Western sensibility: Greek and Roman classics and the Bible. These are sources that European imperial ideology claimed as its Mediterranean legacy (Pratt 10). In fact, Curtis desires these connections so eagerly that he goes so far as to hypothesize that Americans might be the progeny of Anglo-Saxon mixed with Greek (*Nile Notes* 240)!

In my attempt to delineate some of the challenges that the French novelist and the American journalist faced as they panoramically surveyed the exotic spaces and dancing bodies of Egypt in the 1850s, I have discerned a need for constant reassurance for the authority of their gaze and a compulsion to draw from a larger inheritance that they superimpose on the panoramic view. References to Terpsichore and the dance of Greek vases are cases in point. The satisfaction of this need affirms the viewer's subjectivity, and allegiance to Empire and its supremacy. In a succinct, theoretical summation, Ali Behdad theorizes the practice of such panoramic gazing as follows:

> The tendency to have a wide angle of vision is symptomatic of the modern orientalist's fragmentation. Since he can no longer achieve a sense of epistemological totality, he indulges in a scopophilic desire that situates him in a panoptic position from which he can have a panoramic view. The more Flaubert became conscious that he was a tourist passing by, the more he desired an overview of the itinerant space that he never achieved. (58)

Especially when viewing dance, these crises that Behdad describes acquire a renewed urgency. The East may appear like the Bible and the classics but dance jolts the voyeur out of the passivity of "quaint" daily images. Dance also works as "itinerant space" inviting, or rather inducing, the male gaze to experience a different dimension of reality, physical and corporeal space, and sex. Thus, there is a renewed imperative for "epistemological totality" so that the foreign dancing body can be drawn into a familiar zone and the distant to be made local, alleviating some of the anxiety that the contact zone entails. At the same time, familiarizing the dancing body means codifying both the hedonism and the desire invoked by the dance experience, a codification that allows for the transportation of the dance to the drawing rooms of Europe. Although Gustave Flaubert and George William Curtis are not dismayed by Oriental debauchery, they also sense that the bodies they experience in their peregrinations (bodies of land, water, and people) will never accommodate them indigenously. A corollary of this awareness is that these colonized bodies are also capable of mastering the European bourgeois body. Therefore, the dancing body threatens the authority of the European panoramic gaze over the land, sea, interior spaces of buildings, or the native's own body. This panoramic gaze is, in fact, the European's only marker of sovereignty, yet the native body in motion imposes its own control over the imperial subject. And the only comforting "reality" for the imperial subject is the fantasy that, in Bhabha's terminology, the colonized is a fixed "social reality which is at once an 'other' and yet entirely knowable and visible" (70-71). Knowledge of the scriptures, mythology, and the classics constitutes an epistemology that reassures the European subject that he knows "the Orient" as well and may thus violate it. Without these reference points to an assumed European legacy, the panoramic gaze can focus only on horrifying darkness.

Here lies one of the factors that have constructed North and sub-Saharan Africa into such disparate entities in the Western imaginary. Roman ruins lie scattered over North Africa as they do in many parts of Western Europe, including England. Egypt has been charted and studied in relation to Classical Greece and biblical scriptures. If not overwhelmingly Christian, at least North Africa has an organized predominant religion, Islam, and its landscapes seem as familiar as the landscapes of the Bible. However, the panoramic gaze discerned none of these features in the rest of Africa. Imperial nostalgia had neither Roman ruins nor Biblical deserts to predicate itself upon, except an awe-full and menacing primeval past that it feared to look upon or acknowledge.

Flaubert's interpretation of Azizeh's dance poses as a model of these ideologies. Unlike Kuchuk, who comes from Damascus and whose skin is "lighter in coloring than an Arab" (Steegmuller, *Flaubert in Egypt* 114), Azizeh is black, with "frizzy negro hair." In his travel notes, Flaubert affirms that her dancing "is no longer Egypt; it is Negro, African, savage— and wild as the other was formal" (Steegmuller 121). He transcribes her moves but they do not seem familiar from the Greek vases. Under the influence of Azizeh's "wild" interpretation of the dance, Flaubert feels

60

Dismissal
Veiling
Desire:
Kuchuk
Hanem and
Imperial
Masculinity

compelled to revise his earlier impressions of Kuchuk's movement. Now the formality of Kuchuk's dance prevails in his memory of it and serves as a contrast to Azizeh's interpretation, which is, despite its formidable quality, "more expert than Kuchuk's" (121). Flaubert's comparison of the two women is very much about his own self definition. As Robert Young indicates, a prerequisite for Western culture's self definition was racial differentiation. And, Young continues,

> the equation of the white race with civilization (and, as we have seen, of civilization as the cause of whiteness) makes it clear why it was so important during the nineteenth century for the Egyptians not to have been black: this gives a more immediate context and specific rationale for Bernal's argument in *Black Athena* that in the nineteenth century there was a concerted effort to turn the civilization of ancient Egypt from a black one to a white one, than his suggestion of a general conspiracy of European racism. (*Colonial Desire* 95)

Flaubert feels that through scopic conquest and sexual possession he could subdue Kuchuk's power, tame her fancy, and somewhere in the process give form to his own bewildering chaos. Yet, his written accounts indicate only limited success in transcending his gender, cultural, and sexual taboos. Thus, he remains in a position where the initiation he fantasizes remains a remote prospect. The sight of Kuchuk's dancing body is processed through his male conquering gaze, which was established even before he arrived in Egypt and which decided that the body undulating before him was the very site of Orientalism laid open and available. In order to satisfy these needs, the ghaziya's body has to appear like a Mother Earth figure and be a metaphor for the land and also its character. One of the aspects of the dance that has intrigued the Western voyeur is the dancing body's potential to become a vessel for cultural and artistic heritage. With oral tradition being the predominant form for transferring culture through the generations, dance becomes a significant and often highly evocative carrier of religious, social, and sexual aspects of culture. The dancer's body, then, is a palimpsest, recording either an ancient history of art and spirituality or the vulgar ways of the East, with these two extremes often intermingled. Both Flaubert and Curtis subscribe to this dual ideological concept in their attempt to subdue the dancing body and exorcise their fear of it.

Further, Flaubert's awareness of this anticlimactic effect is manifest in the "bitter undertaste" he finds in everything. During the dance he tries hard to decipher the hieroglyphic scripture inscribed in the air by the dancing body, but his gaze is ineffectual because it does not help him read what he sees. George W. Curtis cannot read the dance either, but he is not as vulnerable because he is not interested in being initiated. Instead, he is content to be positioned securely in the seat of his Western status. Looking at the dancer, Flaubert is possessed with a bifurcated desire: to consume her body and also be the body that is consumed by her. His desire for transformation is, at times, overwhelming and manifests itself in his fascination with her jewels, her clothes, and her makeup. His gaze, therefore, discloses at once a will to possess the dancer, a cathexis in the dance as an ecstatic ritual, and an aporia or gap in his understanding.

The ghaziya's dance seems to promise the ultimate meaning of life. However, it fulfills nothing. Instead, the choreography remains like an enigmatic oracle with undecipherable but nevertheless overwhelming meaning. For Flaubert, and likely for others including Curtis who flirted with the sexual prospect, the unique promise offered by sexual union with the dancer fails to inscribe a new trajectory for his life. Flaubert's attempt to conquer these courtesans through ocular and sexual intercourse did not yield the metamorphosis he yearned for, leaving dismissal as the only means to veil unfulfilled desire. Curtis has already dismissed Kuchuk through the constant overdetermined references to her dance as a choreographic reproduction of the past. Of course, Curtis is overtly racist; in his insipid writing style he even proceeds to inane demonstrations of white hegemonic discourse. For example, in his mind, one of the members of Kuchuk's ensemble must be "filially related to a gentle giraffe who had been indiscreet with a hippopotamus" (*Nile Notes* 132). Structuring his story with Kuchuk as *peripeteia* fosters the same kind of discourse. He poses as the protagonist, the hero who meanders into morally perilous territory, brazens out the choreographed threat, annihilates it, and emerges honourable and triumphant: "Farewell Kuchuk! Addio still-eyed dove! Almost thou persuadest me to pleasure" (145).[12]

Even those Europeans who did not experience Kuchuk directly still had some form of intercourse with her. A comparison of Flaubert's recounting of his adventures to Louis Bouilhet with the corresponding content in Flaubert's personal travel journals would merit a study on its own. The effort Flaubert exerts to engage Bouilhet's sexual imagination by recounting his sexual escapades in lurid and explicit terms surpasses mere bravado. In fact, erotic encounters with the East are valuable for Flaubert because they occasion homoerotic descriptions that are decidedly salacious. On these occasions, Flaubert's letters to Bouilhet are

62

Dismissal
Veiling
Desire:
Kuchuk
Hanem and
Imperial
Masculinity

charged with a consuming desire for this apparently very close and beloved male friend. In verbal gestures that call upon Bouilhet, indeed compel him, to relish the experience if only vicariously, Flaubert strikes desiring postures of a very dramatic quality. He is being consumed by longing not only for the East but for Bouilhet as well:

> In my absorption in all those things, *mon pauvre vieux*, you never ceased to be present. The thought of you was like a constant vesicant, inflaming my mind and making its juices flow by adding to the stimulation. I was sorry (the word is weak) that you were not there—I enjoyed it all for myself and for you—the excitement was for both of us, and you came in for a good share, you may be sure. (Steegmuller, *Flaubert in Egypt* 130)

Apparently, Kuchuk becomes the apex of a love triangle that involves Flaubert and Bouilhet. She is used to license a certain form of interaction between them in a medium that she makes safe, paradoxically, by permitting the confirmation of homoerotic attachments. This is a rather exceptional scenario that allows for the colonial project to function as an open closet of male homoerotic bonds in the metropolis itself. In its transgression, the homoeroticism between Bouilhet and Flaubert, validated by the latter's actual Oriental experience, functions as a paradoxical confirmation of the strength of both their male bond and their Europeanness.[13] Eve Kosofsky Sedgwick argues for a continuum that she names "male homosocial desire" (*Between Men* 1), a continuum that has strong implications for the colonial project, which relied greatly on homosocial forms of domination. These forms resulted from a repudiation of homoerotic bonds by the instigation of "homosexual panic":

> Because the paths of male entitlement, especially in the nineteenth century, required certain intense male bonds that were not readily distinguishable from the most reprobated bonds, an endemic and ineradicable state of what I am calling the male homosexual panic became the normal condition of male homosexual entitlement. (*Epistemology of the Closet* 185)

It seems to me that the force of Kuchuk Hanem as a racialized, colonized, and dancing body is such that it dissolves the distinction between reprobated and approved male bonds, thus temporarily suspending what Sedgwick calls homosexual panic. Kuchuk even provides the occasion for celebrating Flaubert's homoerotic desire by being the subject of literature produced with her as the inspiration. Upon their reunion following Flaubert's travels, Bouilhet celebrated the arrival of his long-departed friend by offering him a present of a poem that retold in verse many details from Flaubert's experience in the Orient. The poem was called "Kuchuk Hanem" and was dedicated to Flaubert who received it, Steegmuller informs us, delightedly (*Flaubert and Madame Bovary* 215-16).

Comments that Flaubert sported a "particular brand of romantic misogyny" (Tucker 152), and formulaic statements about Kuchuk as a representation of the Orient that Flaubert wants to possess, have been very popular as component parts of an analysis of the male subject and Eastern dancer dynamic. I return to the scene of Flaubert's first meeting with Kuchuk. Rana Kabbani reacts belligerently to Flaubert's portrayal:

> The onlooker is admitted into the Orient by visual seduction; he encounters the woman in a state of undress, emerging from the intimacy of the bath—in a state of pleasing vulnerability. He is not vulnerable: he is male, presumably in full dress, European, rational (since even when faced with such erotic liability he can still recount the precise details of the apparition quite coolly), and armed with language—he narrates the encounter in a reflective, post-facto narrative; he creates the Orient. (73)

In discussions of Orientalism, such analysis offers a useful tool that has become quite popular because of its formulaic adaptability and analytic possibilities. Yet in its deployment such analysis obliterates Kuchuk Hanem's potential as an agent. Instead, she is fixed with a disposition that the critic assumes for her. Moreover, readings such as Kabbani's somehow restrict venture into further zones of interpretation that encompass the dance and its potency. Instead, we need to think about Kuchuk's kinesthesia as the ultimate marker of difference (gender, racial, and sexual), producing a visceral response in the imperial viewer.

My rather unorthodox pursuit of Kuchuk's evanescent choreographies derives from Marta Savigliano's daring but empowering readings of the tango:

> My interpretations of the tango dance are ambitious, controversial, and too far-reaching. It was precisely this vulnerability, this potential for interpretation, that seemed promising to me. Untamable interpretations (in the sense that they are hard to prove in a positivistic sense) of bodies *performing excessive movement*, despite all the efforts invested in domesticating them, are good signs for a decolonization project. (My emphasis, 13)

Savigliano's declarations encourage me to strive for an assessment of what traditional, ascetic critical activity would prefer to leave untouched. I have taken the risk of focusing on a non-verbal text—choreography—

Dismissal
Veiling
Desire:
Kuchuk
Hanem and
Imperial
Masculinity

that is elusive and evanescent. These efforts have been driven by the bifurcated wish to challenge the usual silence, or even complete disregard, that greets Kuchuk's choreographies in critical work, and to escape the formulaic interpretations that often dominate discussions of this narrative which is invested with such intriguing particularities. Therefore, I have risked indulging in an exploration of how the dancing body influenced the trafficking in emotions and how its choreography was really a necessity to the Empire: a necessity that yielded all the complex responses and approaches that I have tried to analyze. Ultimately, following Savigliano's radical conceptualization of "excessive" movement, Kuchuk's choreographed narratives may conceal signs for undoing the work of colonialism of the Oriental—indeed any—body whose corporeality is trapped in the workings of the imperial heteronormative masculinity. When Said describes these dancers, the allusion to Kuchuk Hanem, and perhaps Azizeh also, is evident. These dancers are "enhanced female types of this legendary, richly suggestive, and associative sort" (*Orientalism* 180). Yet, their special significance for these French writers lies not simply in the dancers' availability and silence but in the complex transformations that their kinesthetic utterances invoke in the imperial subject. A complex matrix of conflicting responses to the dancing body are embedded in Flaubert's biblical reference to the fable of Judith and Holofernes. (I will return to discuss these responses in chapter 4, in relation to Salomé.)

I have lavished attentions on Kuchuk Hanem and her imperial patrons because what took place in her house in Essna was the realization of what Savigliano calls "an imperial erotic relationship with the colonized" (76) and the intricate and powerful evocation of desire and passion and their derivative emotions. However, an imperceptible silence and absence have also pervaded this chapter. I have focused exclusively on heterosexual modes of interaction in dance, ignoring, as critics often do, the male public dancers who were a ubiquitous feature in the nineteenth-century Orient. While in Constantinople, Flaubert watched the performance of dancing boys, a performance that made him overcome by nostalgia for Kuchuk and longing to return to Upper Egypt to be with her (Tsianikas 50, 64). Male Eastern performers demand some long overdue exclusive attention. Their treatment usually varies from complete disregard to hasty or undeveloped comments. Both Joseph Boone (49) and Marjorie Garber complain that in *Orientalism*, Said omits the male dancer and catamite, Hassan el-Balbeissi, whom Flaubert saw before he met Kuchuk and who could also be induced to dance "The Bee," which

Flaubert records and Garber reminds us of (341). As in the encounter with Kuchuk, what took place with Hassan realized "an imperial erotic relationship with the colonized" (Savigliano 76). Flaubert desired to extract from Hassan el-Balbeissi an essence to nurture his bourgeois and voracious desire. In the following chapter, I will examine the intercourse between dancer and viewer but I will focus on the erotic qualities of male dancers who provoked the colonizer's dissipated yearning. Moreover, Gerard de Nerval's account of dancing boys in Cairo will occasion further visitations to the important thematics of ritual and spectacle.

3 / The Dance of Extravagant Pleasures
Male Performers of the Orient and the
Politics of the Imperial Gaze

The dance which followed was of the same description with the singing: it was not the expression of joy, or of gaiety, but of an extravagant pleasure, which made hasty strides toward lasciviousness; and this was the more disgusting, as the performers, all of them of the male sex, presented in the most indecent way scenes which love has reserved for the two sexes in the silence and mystery of the night.

Vivant Denon, *Travels in Upper and Lower Egypt*

Cairo, early June 1834. Edward Lane informs us in a footnote to his chapter on Egypt's public dancers that the city's famous—infamous for many—dancing girls receive the portentous order to abandon their residence in Cairo. The ghawazee are to exile themselves to Upper Egypt with Essna, Qenah, and Aswan designated as their only possible residence options (384). Issuing this edict is Egypt's pasha, Mohamed Ali, an Albanian-born soldier in the Ottoman sultan's army, who came to power in 1805, nominally under Turkish suzerainty. Ali was motivated by a keen commitment to modernize Egypt. Describing his endeavours, Leila Ahmed underlines the emphasis he placed on utilizing resources and passing reforms that would ultimately secure economic and administrative independence for Egypt:

> Intent upon making Egypt independent, Muhammad Ali set about modernizing his army and increasing revenues. He introduced agricultural, administrative, and educational reforms and attempted to establish industries, his initiatives in these areas giving impetus to economic, intellectual, cultural, and educational developments important to women. (131)

67   Notes to chapter 3 are on page 208.

68

The Dance of
Extravagant
Pleasures:
Male
Performers
of the Orient
and the
Politics of
the Imperial
Gaze

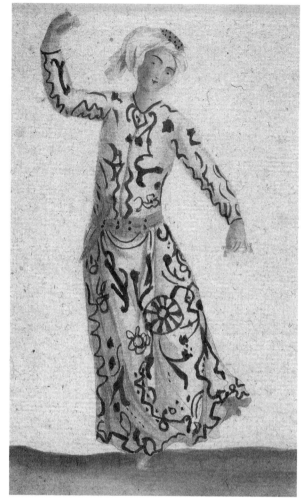

Photo of a hand-painted copper plate engraving from 1760-1780, representing a dancing boy playing clappers. A dancing boy was called koçek which means "little camel colt." He is in a yellow robe with a sash, a dagger, and a turban. Most dancing boys came from non-Turkish cultures of the Ottoman Empire. (Caption by Elizabeth Artemis Mourat. Photo courtesy of the private collection of Elizabeth Artemis Mourat.)

Examined in the context of colonial discourse, a non-Western ruler's ambition to "modernize" his "Oriental" state implies—almost invariably to me, a Cypriot who has seen it happen in his own country—some sort of genuflection to the imposition of the technological and cultural superiority of Western Europe. Modernization further indicates a willingness to allow, even invite, colonial influence, involvement, or dependence.

69

The Dance of
Extravagant
Pleasures:
Male
Performers
of the Orient
and the
Politics of
the Imperial
Gaze

Indeed, he proceeds to make his reforms following the propositions of European advisors brought especially to lend their expertise in constructing a new, Westernized, industrialized, and fortified Egypt. Nonetheless, as Leila Ahmed indicates, "in their immediate impact, both Western economic advances and Muhammad Ali's policies adversely affected some women, particularly lower-class urban and rural women" (131). However, neither here nor elsewhere does Ahmed make reference to the dancers of Cairo, so their social position and the nature of their profession remain undiscussed and, therefore, completely absent from an otherwise thorough and well-researched project. What emerges from Ahmed's (problematic) silence on the issue is that the fate of the ghawazee became entangled in Mohamed Ali's "eagerness to acquire the technologies of Europe, which was an important catalyst" (133) in Egyptian affairs of this time. The edict that banished dancers and courtesans to Upper Egypt was, perhaps, a measure to alleviate the pasha's embarrassment at his country's popular arts and customs, as Morroe Berger suggests, and to appease religious authorities: Mohamed Ali "became ashamed, I suppose, not only of his domain's economic backwardness but of its popular arts as well. Partly because of the bad impression they made on foreigners and partly because of pressure from religious leaders, Muhammad Ali barred the public dancing girls from the Cairo area in 1834" (30). Berger's syntax here is ambiguous: it seems to make the disturbing suggestion that the Egyptian leader's domain was indeed economically "backward," an interesting enactment of the kind of imperialism that the pasha had to contend with in the early nineteenth century. Indeed, if shame was Mohamed Ali's motivation, then his edict relied on an attempt to shift the territory of these artists' influence away from the bustling, cosmopolitan metropolis of Cairo.[1]

However, I am inclined to believe that more than religious authorities, the principal motive for banishing the ghawazee was to appease the Europeans, since the poor impression that many foreign visitors claimed to have about the dancers had become legendary. Vivant Denon's 1798 description of female dancers is one of the early examples of imperial dismay over the production of Oriental kinesthetic art:

They were seven in number. Two of them began dancing, while the others sung, with an accompaniment of castanets, in the shape of cymbals, and of the size of a crown piece. The movement they displayed in striking them against each other gave infinite grace to their fingers and wrists. At the commencement the dance was voluptuous: it soon after became lascivious,

70

The Dance of
Extravagant
Pleasures:
Male
Performers
of the Orient
and the
Politics of
the Imperial
Gaze

and expressed, in the grossest and most indecent way the giddy transports of the passions. The disgust which this spectacle excited was heightened by one of the musicians … who, at the moment when the dancers gave the greatest freedom to their wanton gestures and emotions, with the stupid air of a clown in a pantomime, interrupted by a loud burst of laughter the scene of intoxication which was to close the dance. (232-33)

By 1845, James Augustus St. John voiced a generally accepted opinion that "many travellers affect to have been much disgusted by the performances of the Ghazeeyeh" (*Egypt and Nubia* 270). In fact, even though the Orientalist (as Edward Said uses the term) sources do not make the point explicitly, some important facts point to Mohamed Ali's European advisors as the main agent in securing the prohibition. For example, the very economics of the dancers' occupation manifest their indispensability. Again, according to Lane, because of their popularity the ghawazee were numerous and enjoyed very high incomes, thus making a significant contribution to the Cairo-area income tax revenue (Lane 388). Apparently, following their exile, the sultan had to levy heavier personal taxes to compensate for revenue sacrificed to moral zeal. However, apart from the economics of the situation, the ghawazee were significant as an evidently established cultural institution. Their performances were considered essential at celebrations such as wedding parties, festivals, and circumcision ceremonies. Clearly, their artistic contribution to such events must have been important.[2] Directly associated with the Western gaze's effect was the opprobrium perceived to mark the dancers' performances, which scandalized some travellers and stimulated their negative accounts. In other words, the lasciviousness of the dance is an attribute that came to exist during scopic intercourse with the Western gaze.

Apparently, following Mohamed Ali's edict and the departure of large numbers of dancers and courtesans to Upper Egypt, the Cairo scene became inundated with khawals, dancing boys called gink, or çengi and koçek in Turkish. Rather amusingly, the ghawazee were sent away so as not to offend morals, yet as Morroe Berger informs us, the male dancers who came to prevail in their wake presented an even more relentless challenge to Western mores: "the number of male Oriental dancers increased, and they, as Flaubert found, were often more audacious and salacious than the girls. The male dancers were already famous before the banishment of the *almées*" (30).[3] These are enticing pieces of information that titillate, yet undermine Berger's intentions to offer an objective and constructive appraisal of Middle Eastern dance. This is clearly a moment

71

The Dance of
Extravagant
Pleasures:
Male
Performers
of the Orient
and the
Politics of
the Imperial
Gaze

when his article lapses into Orientalist banter that fails to offer an honest or engaging interpretation of male dancing in nineteenth-century Egypt. But I am still intrigued by the question of who exactly found the khawals more audacious and salacious. By whose standards were their performances more "lascivious" than the women's and to what extent did the performers' gender affect the Western tourists' assessment?

My purpose in this chapter is to examine the dynamics of Western interaction with the Middle Eastern male dancing body and the ways in which the questions of audience and moral standards affect the larger issues of colonial interaction and the colonial discourse that resulted from it. A force that propels this project derives from my personal involvement in Middle Eastern dance and my effort to deal with the variety of responses to my performance. Participating in an art form that, in the minds of most people in the West, is exclusively female, I often have to contend with attitudes both from audiences and dance instructors. That is, most attempts to recuperate modern belly dance have relied on reconstructions of this dance as the remnant of women's fertility rites associated with primeval goddess worship.[4] For some decades now these views have circulated as confident convictions developed under the rubric of feminism but regarded with mistrust within feminism itself, although performance of this dance can be, and is for many, a valuable service to women's liberation.[5] While this service is entirely agreeable, such a reconstruction of Oriental dance is nonetheless so widespread that it is not merely part of the West, in the geographical and cultural specificities that define the West today (primarily North America and Western Europe) but has established itself internationally. I think that globalizing the "femininity" of this art is disconcerting because it predicates itself on certain romantic notions that have distorted crucial aspects of this dance's traditions. For example, constructing modern Oriental dance as a female fertility ritual silences the widespread custom of male dancers in the East. Moreover, the legacy of colonial dynamics and Western imperialism plays itself out in those individual European and North American instructors and performers of contemporary interpretations of Oriental dance. Many see themselves in the role of "rescuers" of this tradition. Yet, in this rescue operation they fail or refuse to acknowledge the history of colonialism and the biases or privilege that their Western position bestows upon them. Especially problematic is the conviction that if it weren't for dance schools and instructors in North America, this dance would not have survived into our present time. This is a much-encountered belief among

72

*The Dance of
Extravagant
Pleasures:
Male
Performers
of the Orient
and the
Politics of
the Imperial
Gaze*

the belly dance community. (I will return to discuss this disconcerting phenomenon in the concluding chapter.)

I do not mean to reassess male involvement in Middle Eastern public dancing with the ultimate purpose of reclaiming male dominance (ubiquitous in most aspects of society and art anyway) in this artistic tradition. Such a purpose would be extreme and even spurious. Instead, I wish to explore gender politics whose multifarious complexity emerges mainly from native kinesthetic expression before the imperial gaze. This gaze is, in fact, the main province of my investigation with my interest extending to the female performers as well as the male, since the dynamics of the female performance are inextricably linked with those of the male, especially in the imperial context. The processes that moulded Western attitudes towards dancers in the Middle East in the latter age of European imperialist and colonial expansion have effectively defined contemporary attitudes as well. Regarding these perspectives Anthony Shay has been urging us to recognize significant complexities in the politics that determine dance. These attitudes, Shay argues, are not the prerogative of "foreign" Western audiences but also "native elites"—those individuals from colonized countries where imperialism has taken deep roots. These are people, artists among them, who had and continue to have vested interests in replicating the Western world view and perpetuating the colonial project mainly, but not exclusively, because of economic investments or political interests.

One example of this kind of imperial interference in indigenous traditions has figured in the introduction to this chapter. The ghawazee were banned because, under the Western gaze, the quality of their art was questioned, thus turning their dancing into cultural embarrassment. If Berger is indeed accurate in assessing the influence of Egyptian religious leaders and European advisors in Egypt, then both these factions shared concerns that seem to have coincided in effecting this development that pushed the dancers' cultural activity into the space that Anne McClintock defines as "anachronistic." Under the new measures for the implementation of a "new" Egypt, the dancers become the "inherently atavistic, living archive of the primitive archaic" (McClintock 41), incompatible with progress. Europeans moved into Egypt with their bourgeois moral pretensions serving as a fulcrum to implement policies that would civilize, educate, and refine its "savage" inhabitants. These pretensions became, in fact, a perfect means for policing human behaviour abroad. Of course, such intentions were unsettled by the European experience of polymor-

73

*The Dance of
Extravagant
Pleasures:
Male
Performers
of the Orient
and the
Politics of
the Imperial
Gaze*

phous "Eastern perversity," which fuelled the efforts for reform and set in motion the circular process required to sustain assumed imperial responsibility. Eastern excess and its resistance to representation, let alone containment and control, came to be embodied in the Middle Eastern dancer's performance. Both the physical embodiment and the theoretical implications of the dance became a metaphor for much of what the West perceived as "Oriental." By physical embodiment I am referring to the actual dance moves, which provided a somatic articulation unlike any that Western eyes were used to or could culturally accept as public spectacle. Choreographies of Middle Eastern public performers, male and female, largely consisted of suggestive contortions: writhing, undulating, swaying the body with side twists, isolated muscle quivering, and rhythmically elaborate hip articulations (Azizeh's "furious jerking of the hips" [Steegmuller, *Flaubert in Egypt* 122]). The theoretical implications of such choreographies for the Western spectators were overwhelming, as Flaubert and Curtis's travel accounts illustrate in relation to Kuchuk. Europeans' conventional expectations of corporeal, gendered behaviour were contravened dramatically. Generations of cultural dogma confined the hips, shoulders, and the lumbar region to a controlled attitude that signalled a state of embarrassed silence. By contrast, in Middle Eastern dance these body parts acquired an expression enunciating a carnal sensuality and desire even to the uninitiated, unaccustomed, and undiscerning European eye.

Viewed as text, a choreographic sequence of Oriental dance spelled out a hieroglyphics of uninhibited sexual desire and wantonness. As Lady Mary Wortley Montague writes from Adrianople in 1717:

> This dance was very different from what I had seen before. Nothing could be more artful, or more proper to raise *certain ideas*. The tunes so soft!— The motions so languishing!—accompanied with pauses and dying eyes! half-falling back, and then recovering themselves in so artful a manner, that I am very positive the coldest and most rigid prude upon earth, could not have looked upon them without thinking of *something not to be spoken of*. (163)

Evidently, Montague's text revels in the erotic posturing of the dance. The details she chooses to describe gesture strongly toward an exhibition of sexuality that clearly challenges her racial and social identification. Nevertheless, Montague's assessment of the dance is kindly devoid of vehement disapproval or emphasis on excess and lasciviousness. This generosity is perhaps predictable if one considers that her views were radical for her

74

*The Dance of
Extravagant
Pleasures:
Male
Performers
of the Orient
and the
Politics of
the Imperial
Gaze*

time, marking a departure from the stereotypical representations of Oriental society instituted by travel writers who preceded her. Drawing from her special involvement with Turkish female society, Montague challenged and criticized these earlier writers' published misconceptions and sought to represent a revised view of Turkish culture. Nonetheless, in accordance with the norms of her time, she brackets overt sexuality from the performance of the dance, its manifestation confined to silence— "not to be spoken of."[6]

If a "lady" traveller had to confine sexuality to the unspeakable, European men had equivalent difficulties. To the average Western male gaze, Middle Eastern dance epitomized the aberrance believed to be innate in Eastern culture as a whole and dictated the assumption of a detached, critical stance. As an othered topos, the dancer's body was a site too fluid and evasive, articulating a meaning that was deemed unreachable when its obvious significations were too threatening to dwell upon. Dance was, therefore, impossible to naturalize or institutionalize even when deciphered as desire. Desire, in fact, was the domain of potency since, quite often, the male Western spectators felt themselves hovering in that perilous space just past the edge of their imperial virtue and just before the surrender to the semiotics of the dance, which invoked the inexorable urge to possess the dancer's body.

Lane's description of the ghawazee in *The Modern Egyptians* is quite revealing of this profound ambivalence towards the Eastern dancer as a trope of the East in general:

> The Ghawazee perform, unveiled, in the public streets, even to amuse the rabble. Their dancing has little of elegance; its chief peculiarity being a very rapid vibrating motion of the hips, from side to side. They commence with a degree of decorum; but soon, by more animated looks, by a more rapid collision of their castanets of brass, and by increased energy in every motion, they exhibit a spectacle exactly agreeing with the descriptions which Martial and Juvenal have given of the performances of the female dancers of Gades. (384)

Gades, otherwise known as Cadiz, was a Phoenician colony and subsequently a Roman conquest. It enjoyed a great reputation for its dancers who were celebrated by several Roman writers. Juvenal described dancers who "sink to the ground and quiver with applause ... a stimulus for languid lovers, nettles to whip rich men to live" (qtd. in Buonaventura 43). Martial, a Roman satirist, records a special characteristic of these dancers' moves in a dinner invitation that details exotic pleasures which his guest

75

*The Dance of
Extravagant
Pleasures:
Male
Performers
of the Orient
and the
Politics of
the Imperial
Gaze*

will not experience: "nor will girls from naughty Gades, endlessly pruri-ent, vibrate their wanton thighs with sweet trembling."[7] Apart from exhibiting his erudition, Lane is also reiterating the romantic notion of the Orient as a seamless continuation with a distant past and presenting it, in effect, as a rich kaleidoscope of primeval scenes unfolding before the European gaze. Moreover, his brief yet apathetic analysis of the dance is an unpersuasive attempt to feign a lack of interest. Further in the same chapter he betrays his fascination and disdain: "I need scarcely add that these women are the most abandoned of the courtesans of Egypt. Many of them are extremely handsome; and most of them are richly dressed. Upon the whole, I think they are the finest women in Egypt" (386).

The availability and promise of these women are the very qualities identified with the East and paradoxically the qualities that generate anxiety in the Western traveller. This anxiety arises from a complex matrix of responses. In travellers' accounts, there is a feeling of being implicated in Eastern depravity through the gaze itself, a guilt obfuscated by the often repressed desire for the dancer, and the perceived pressure to per-form in response to the Oriental performance. As I suggest in the previ-ous chapter, the argument which defines the Oriental subject as the abject object of the Occidental gaze has to be reconsidered in light of the agency of the Oriental dancer's body and choreography, both of which provoke a complex interaction with the viewer. In discussing a video clip by the female Afro-American pop group TLC, Susan Foster addresses pre-cisely what I infer from the ghawazee's performance:

> The dancers repeatedly invite the camera and, implicitly, the viewer toward them, gesturing the body's sensuality and desire. Masterfully they rebuff, refocus, and reorient the gaze so as to control access to intimacy. Standing firm, they mock the objectification of the female body. Slipping deftly out from under the gaze's scrutiny, they illuminate pathways of desire whose directionality and accessibility they have crafted. By chore-ographing such a complex relationship to the gaze, these women artists embody the tense dynamism of their identities as Afro-American and feminist, as members of an oppressed and marginalized social group, and as leaders in an international avant-garde aesthetic. ("Choreographies of Gender" 16)

Albeit without the advanced technological means of contemporary video-clip creation, the ghawazee's choreography also gestures the body's sen-suality and sexual promise. Masterfully, their body rebuffs, refocuses, and reorients the gaze "so as to control access to intimacy." Especially in this

76

*The Dance of
Extravagant
Pleasures:
Male
Performers
of the Orient
and the
Politics of
the Imperial
Gaze*

dance idiom where the moves have to be isolated, this isolation takes the place of the camera focus. Through deft moves executed under the male gaze's scrutiny, the dancers "illuminate pathways of desire whose directionality and accessibility they have crafted." By choreographing such a complex relationship to the Western gaze, the ghawazee embody their own tense dynamism and potency as well as that of the East. Therefore, they must be banished if order is to prevail over sexual anarchy in the emerging, modernized, Westernized Egypt.

It was through this very complex configuration of contraries—desire and disavowal, control and abandon—that the female dancers "increasingly came to be fetishized into an isolated female sign of the Orient's erotic and passionate potential" (Lewis 173). There is an imperative in this sign: the ghawazee had to be contained in this image so that passion, an imperial emotion projected onto the native performer, could proceed with its circulation and yield desire (Flaubert's and Curtis's narratives, discussed in the previous chapter, delineate this process). The ghawazee became the sign on account of their sex. If European Orientalists resisted them, then the contestant for this sign would be male dancers, who were perceived to engender further vilification of European sensibility and morals. Passion and desire engaged in their magnetic courtship dance on the colonial field would cease to be heterosexual, turning, instead,

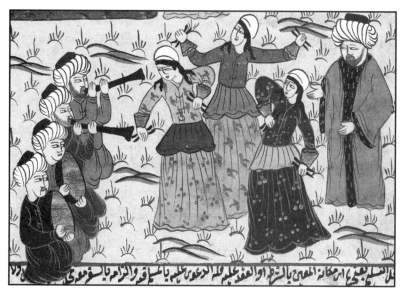

Ottoman miniature painting of dancing boys. (Courtesy of the private collection of Elizabeth Artemis Mourat.)

homoerotic. In the eyes of travellers, male performance was similar to the ghawazee's in technique and style except that their gender posed a far more formidable threat to European sexual ethics. What is important to point out, however, is that these male dancers were indispensable as well as threatening. Their dance set in motion those mechanisms that regulated the emotional capital of the Empire. Thus, they engendered anxiety and fear framed by desire.

The Poetics of Male Dancing

Male dancers' presence and popularity, not only in Egypt but also over the entire Middle East and as far as Central Asia, had a long and strongly felt presence. Their survival, however, has depended largely on the narratives of Western visitors to the East. In Turkey at least, the "early Turkish sources offer little information" on dancers (male and female) because "dancing was regarded by many writers of the past as an improper and wicked sport, especially when indulged in by professional women and boys" (Metin And 138). A selection of these narratives might assist in envisioning their activities and bodies as sites that have generated sexual meanings for the Empire. It is especially significant that these sites helped hypostatize the European man's heteronormativity.

As early as 1675, Dr John Covel's diaries describe "a delicate lovely boy, of about 10 yeares old," and, dancing with him, "a lusty handsome man (about 25) both Turkes. They acceded all the roguish lascivious postures conceived with that strange ingenuity of silent ribaldry" (*Early Voyages* 214). Although Covel's account of these dancers is succinct and circumspect, it firmly sets the tone of ambivalence. As it emerges here, their choreography, enacted in "lascivious postures," supposedly displays an innate, intelligent, and inspired vulgarity—a near oxymoron that aptly conveys the seduction but also the indecency embodied by the male dancer of the East in the eyes of the bourgeois traveller.[8] Vivant Denon was less subtle in his disapproval. In 1810, Lord Byron and John Hobhouse enjoyed performances by transvestite boys in the coffeehouses of Galata, a Constantinople suburb famous for its tavernas. Apparently Hobhouse found the demonstration "beastly" (Garber 418) but Byron's reaction is unrecorded (Murray 24). Dating from the same period (the first quarter of the nineteenth century) is Lady Augusta Hamilton's account of these singing and dancing boys, with its delightful and appetizing details. She writes in 1822, "they are dressed like girls, and accompany words adapted

78

The Dance of
Extravagant
Pleasures:
Male
Performers
of the Orient
and the
Politics of
the Imperial
Gaze

to the purpose, with wanton looks and gestures, which will often so please their employers, that they will almost cover the boys' faces with ducats, sticking them on with their spittle; and the boys, in their turn, have the dexterity, in the course of the dance, to slide them almost imperceptibly into their pockets" (49).[9] In the early nineteenth century, fights in these coffeehouses broke out frequently among the Janissaries, the sultan's soldiers, who were fervent admirers and competed for the attention of these boys (who were also known as koçek). According to Thijs Janssen, "it was generally assumed that koçek [another name for çengi] could be buggered. This explains much of the excitement of the male spectators, many of whom courted the koçek" (84-85). The period that Hamilton writes about, approximately the time when Byron was in the taverns of Galata, must have seen the apogee of the male dancers' popularity.

Another Western source testifying to the popularity of dancing boys, but also pointing out their salaciousness, forms part of Eugene Schuyler's journey through Turkistan. Schuyler was the United States consul in Russia, an office he held before he embarked on his travels in central Asia in 1867. In places he visited, especially in Uzbekistan, he found that Mohammedan prudery did not allow women to dance in public, therefore their role came to be fulfilled by "boys and youths" called batchas. "The moral tone of the society of Central Asia is scarcely improved by the change" (70), he adds. He proceeds to give an account of their enthusiastic reception by audiences and their esteemed status as artists:

> These batchas ... are a recognized institution throughout the whole of the settled portions of Central Asia, though they are most in vogue in Bukhara, and the neighbouring Samarkand. Batchas are as much respected as the greatest singers and artistes are with us. Every movement they make is followed and applauded, and I have never seen such breathless interest as they excite, for the whole crowd seems to devour them with their eyes, while their hands beat time to every step. (70)

A few paragraphs later, in an attempt to fulfill his responsibility as an informed exponent of the exotic culture, he makes what seems like an honest and serious attempt to assess responsibly these boys' art for his readers: "The dances, so far as I was able to judge, were by no means indecent, though they were often very lascivious" (71). The oddness of this comment lies in the distinction Schuyler expects his readers to make between decency and lasciviousness. If the dancers were decent, how then were they lascivious? Whatever the referents are for the terms, what is important to note is the anxiety and the excitement that generates their use and the anxiety and the excitement that this use in turn generates.

Edward Lane is also graphic but not as elaborate when providing information on the dancing boys on the Egyptian scene, especially Cairo:

> As they personate women, their dances are exactly of the same description as those of the Ghawazee; and are, in like manner, accompanied by the sounds of castanets: but, as if to prevent their being thought to be really females, their dress is suited to their *unnatural* profession; being partly male, and partly female: it chiefly consists of a tight vest, a girdle, and a kind of petticoat. Their general appearance, however, is more feminine than masculine: they suffer the hair of the head to grow long, and generally braid it, in the manner of the women; the hair on the face, when it begins to grow, they pluck out; and they imitate the women also in applying kohl and henna to their eyes and hands. In the streets, when not engaged in dancing, they often even veil their faces; not from shame, but merely to affect the manners of women. *They are often employed, in preference to the Ghawazee*, to dance before a house, or in its court, on the occasion of a marriage-fête, or the birth of a child, or a circumcision; and frequently perform at public festivals. There is in Cairo, another class of male dancers, young men and boys, whose performances, dress, and general appearance are almost exactly similar to those of the Khawals; but who are distinguished by a different appellation, which is "Gink"; a term that is Turkish, and has a vulgar signification which aptly expresses their character. They are generally Jews, Armenians, Greeks, and Turks. (My emphasis, 389)

Having committed himself to providing an account of the manners and customs of the Egyptian people, Lane acts as if he has little choice but to include this description of the khawals. He does not spend many lines on them, his chapter focusing mostly on the ghawazee even though it is entitled "Public Dancers." Apparently, he finds their numbers small enough that he prefers to dedicate more space in his account to the more numerous ghawazee. Noteworthy, however, are his own comments on the demand for the khawals. He tells us that they are often employed and frequently perform at public festivals. In a subsequent chapter on private festivities, he mentions that in the morning after a child's birth, "two or three of the dancing men called Khawals, or two or three Ghazeeyehs, dance in front of the house, or in the court" (509). Male and female performers are, in other words, interchangeable and sometimes the males are even preferred as he mentions in the lengthy passage above. Nonetheless, there is a note of discomfort regarding the effeminate dress and cus-

80

The Dance of
Extravagant
Pleasures:
Male
Performers
of the Orient
and the
Politics of
the Imperial
Gaze

toms of the khawals and an obvious tone of disapproval in labelling their profession "unnatural." Lane's closing remark on "the vulgar signification" of Gink, a remark that indicates a certain discomfort, seems to allude to these dancers' explicit availability for sexual hire (as Stephen Murray notes in "The Will Not to Know" 46, n24). Obviously, the Janissaries' enthusiasm over the dancing boys was not as openly shared, if felt at all, by either Lane or the majority of travellers to the Middle East. Sodomy, as interpreted in the West, forced the Occidental tourist to face a challenge that is often discursively construed as unsuspected or unforeseen and is, therefore, insidious as well as scandalous for the imperial subject.

On this same issue of homosexual sex, Charles S. Sonnini, a former engineer in the French navy and an intrepid traveller and naturalist, pauses in his narrative to lament:

> The unnatural passion which some Thracian women punished by slaying Orpheus, who had entertained it, the inconceivable inclination which has dishonoured the Greeks and the Persians of antiquity, constitute this delight, or, more properly speaking, the infamy of Egyptians. It is not for women that their amorous sonnets are composed; it is not to them that they lavish tender caresses; no; other objects inflame their desires.... Such depravation, which to the shame of polished nations is not unknown to them, is universally spread in Egypt. (163)

This is the passage written by a man who seems eager to join any army of enraged Maenads to lay vengeful hands on male flesh tainted by homoerotic pleasure, this unnameable and unnatural vice. Reading the same passage, Joseph Boone finds that "a note of hysteria" infiltrates this narrative (51), a note that is remarkably strident. "Part of the horror," Boone correctly observes, "is that this 'inconceivable appetite' 'is not altogether unknown' to civilized Europe: if the Egyptian vice knows no class ('rich and poor are equally infected by it'), can it be expected to respect the boundaries of colonizer and colonized?" (52).

Particularly in the context of dance, this hysteria is exacerbated by more disconcerting and anxiety-provoking images. If the ghawazee provoke the Western male visitor with a voyeuristic spectacle that upsets his moral pretensions, the encounter with the khawals forces him into that most awkward and discomfiting space between genders where he realizes a particularly tantalizing desire. Enclasped in this space, the imperial subject is impelled to confront a liminal identity, one that becomes the most vivid, shameless, and lurid embodiment of his taboos. The apparently great popularity of these performers (a popularity that spanned long his-

torical periods) exacerbated the "delicate" position of the Western viewers. Even if they felt any enthusiasm over the koçek, the khawals, or the
batchas, their enthusiasm had to be closeted in the narrative. For example, Sonnini even finds it impossible to name the act, as if to deny it entry
into discourse. As a result, homosexual desire or its concomitant acts are
present only through unnameability and silence, looming over the Egypt-
ian/Oriental domain, even though they are "not unknown" to civilized,
European nations.

Ironically, it is not only the European narratives that convey strong
phobias as they become overwhelmed by the lurid spectacle of male performers. Writers from within the traditions also display these familiar
attitudes. Metin And, a Turkish researcher writing about the dance traditions of Anatolia, details the male dancers' artistic contribution and
its impact on their admirers like this:

> Their manner and dress were suited to their unnatural profession; being
> partly male, and partly female, they were so loved and lauded by their
> audiences that many poets sang their praises in verse. They praised their
> physical beauty as well as their skill in their art. One of the most notable
> poets was the famous poet, Enderunlu Fazil. His Defteri Aşk (meaning
> "Book of Love") contains 170 couplets praising the beauty and skill of
> the celebrated eighteenth century dancing boy, Çingene Ismail. His *Çeng-
> iname*, a book about the famous dancing boys of the early nineteenth cen-
> tury, gives the names and stage names of forty-five performers. (141)

And's passage provides a good example of the frustrations involved when
one wants to reconstruct an epistemology of male performers in the Orient. Their reception was so ambivalent, apparently in their own culture
as well, that adequate understanding of the contradictions in the sources
themselves is difficult. Two pages before the passage quoted above, And
talks of the dearth of references to these dancers in Turkish literature
because of their low social esteem. At this point, he tells us that there have
been Turkish poets praising the male dancers' every aspect. Being a Turkish scholar, Metin And could have made a valuable contribution by focusing on this apparently significant institution of Turkish culture. He could
have provided some quotations from these poets and a discussion of their
work in order to clarify the social changes that elapsed between the
silence of the "early" authors and the early nineteenth century, when a
Turkish poet exalted the dancing boys. But he doesn't. Finally, the opening of the passage here, "Their manner and dress ... being partly male, and
partly female" comes from that much-quoted passage from Lane that is

The Dance of
Extravagant
Pleasures:
Male
Performers
of the Orient
and the
Politics of
the Imperial
Gaze

also quoted in this section. Not only does And leave this reference uncited, as if it forms part of his own text, he also allows it to challenge the meaning of the rest of his paragraph. In other words, he does not explain the paradox involved in an "unnatural profession" attracting such love and admiration.

Similarly, Kemal Özdemir in his *Oriental Belly Dance* posits with alarming confidence that modern performances of this dance are all about heterosexual intercourse. He writes that "Oriental belly dance is the artistic expression of man's innate instinct to reproduce reflected in the female's rhythmic movements," and that "when the dancer turns her back to the onlooker and swings her hips, she sends a message which can be interpreted as the call for copulation" (64). Shocking as they may seem (and at several moments quite offensive), Özdemir's interpretations try to make sense of the dance in terms of heterosexuality, while his sexism secures a safe passage for the project in the patriarchal mainstream. Therefore, his chapters on the çengi and the koçek are decidedly at odds with the general attitude, tone, and purpose of the book. Like Metin And, Kemal Özdemir seems keen on relating this part of Turkish artistic tradition (in fact, his report on the dancing boys is elaborate) but does not seem to recognize the paradoxes that his position evokes. The çengi are said to be very popular female entertainers, famous and beloved for their skilled dancing. "Young men looking for enjoyment and well-to-do womanizers clustered around such houses but it was only very seldom that chengis had a good time with men…. In short, Ottoman chengis were renowned for their unabashed lesbianism" (37-38). Similarly, the great appeal and popularity of the male dancers, the koçek, emerge in Özdemir's references to Evliya Çelebi, a traveller who offers an erotic and doting depiction of some of the dancing boys: "curly-haired, doe-eyed and long-lashed Dimitraki, Neferaki and Yanaki of [the island of] Chios are the best köchecks [*sic*] who have set Istanbul on fire and spent the treasures of many an admirer, causing them to fall prey to deep poverty" (54-56). At one moment, Özdemir seems to attribute the koçeks' irresistible charm to the perfection of their drag, suggesting that spectators loved them because the dancers' true sex eluded them:

> They sometimes danced fully dressed like women whereby no one could tell the difference between the sexes, and in such cases, the air would overflow with "oh's" and "ah's" and the wind of lust would take hold of everyone. These beautiful male coquettes drove men crazy with their seductive sighs and oriental dance. (59)

Of course, dance moves are potent because they conceal sexual codes. Özdemir's overtly heterosexual analysis, however, offers no relief for the unspeakability and taboo of sex, while female sexuality is vulgarized in his interpretation that is accompanied by a pandemonium of photos depicting voluptuous dancers in a variety of postures (one caption reads, "a [male] spectator dreaming of something private" 147). Sadly too, his information on the male dancers (and the female çengi) appears like precious, gleaming fragments against a backdrop that continuously strives to distort, obscure, or blur them.[10]

To conclude this section on the poetics of male dancing, I will turn to another Turkish writer whose travel narrative contributes intriguing dance scenes with male performers. The author is Irfan Orga, who travelled in Turkey possibly in the late 1930s although the date is not specified. Orga observes scenes of Turkish life with a gaze that is native but inflected by a certain morality that raises questions about his cultural influences and the audience he imagines for his narrative. The communities that Orga depicts during his travels in *The Caravan Moves On* have very set notions of decency and respectability and strictly observe social codes and hierarchies. Marriage is often not simply expected but imposed, the women have to be virgins before marriage, the signs that denote manhood and womanhood are clear and undisputed. However, he describes a brief but overwhelming incident that makes a crucial intervention in these traditions. While visiting Konya and the surrounding region, Orga stays with Hikmet Bey, a powerful landowner of great influence and together they visit an isolated farm owned by Hikmet Bey. At the farm, following a heavy dinner and generous consumption of *raki*, a locally produced alcoholic drink, Orga narrates a fascinating scene of lush eroticism that raises the spectre of homosexual sex and the homoerotics of male performance. The singer who provides the first part of after-dinner entertainment is a slender young man of about twenty, with a womanish figure, who sings in a low and sweet voice that "teases" Hikmet Bey's emotions. When a young boy dances, however, the scene turns into an unexpected ritual that invokes a confounding pathos:

> For a few moments the boy stood slackly, but one felt the ripple of excitement that went through the watching men. For a little longer the boy timed his movements against the beat of the music, little hesitant movements that were suggestive of young amorous limbs. Then he began to dance, carefully, painstakingly—almost clumsily—keeping in perfect time with the quickening music. His smooth young face was as blank as a sleep-

walker's. He weaved a pattern with his feet, but his mind was somewhere else. His artistry was superb, for the movements of his body and the fluttering hands portrayed unmistakably a young girl's first reluctance to physical love, her gradual desire to experience it, finally her surrender. (51)

It is clear in the description that the sensuality of this moment is overwhelming for almost every man present: "Men sat in rapt attention.... The half-darkness was rapacious and secretive and all eyes were directed to the boy who swayed in moaning rapture, his dark shadow leaping up the wall behind him—monstrous, gigantic" (51). The fascination of the moment is clearly audible in the compelling ecstasy to which many of the men surrender, as the author tells us. The experience incites in Orga thoughts about the mysteries of life, love, and death, and the inevitability of fate. More importantly, however, the experience with the dancer intimates a kind of queer (both in its sense of "strange" and "homosexual") desiring fulfilled by a pained, ecstatic consummation in which Orga does not indulge. Both these processes, the desiring and the course of consummation, seem unattached to societal structures and established institutions that the author comments on in the narrative.

It would almost seem as if we as readers are invited to perceive this scene of dance and choreographed sexual and spiritual ecstasy as a site left deliberately empty so it can accommodate a kind of love and eroticism that approximate mainstream, acceptable modes but are not quite mainstream or acceptable. As the author puts it in the passage I quote above, the dancer is superb not as a male dancer but because he is like a young girl about to be deflowered; his act is the same as a girl's—but not quite. Nonetheless, it is fascinating how, for the others present, this site seems sacred in an almost metaphysical sense. Orga does not surrender to the seduction of the dancer even though, as he puts it, "he singled me out for his attentions, standing so close in front of me that I was aware of the little pulse beating in his throat and his head outlined in flaring candlelight" (50-51). The profundity and profanity of this enchanting moment touch him deeply. Before his reader, however, he claims to remain sober enough to check his rapture and avoid falling into the trap of such "low" passions:

> I found the experience of that night both moving and chilling, an experience so primitive that it could not fail to stir the blood, yet so expressive of man's lower nature, so imprisoning, that one felt brushed by the Devil himself. The room was full of *raki* fumes, of sweating humanity and the queer acrid odour of the copulations of older men. To stagger out to

the sweet night air was a form of relief, for unless one has lost one's senses in drink it is impossible not to be appalled by licentiousness. (52)

In my estimation, the author employs the trope of "primitiveness" in this narrative not so much because of its explanatory potential. The term "primitive" carries an ideological charge that allows Orga to disguise the melancholy that is associated with the intense desiring manifest in this moment, and which has marked his emotions deeply. Of course, this disguise is (perhaps deliberately) diaphanous since in the closing image of his chapter he gazes at his own spellbound reflection: "the moon was high in the sky, infinitely remote, symbol of men's dreams. Trees stood out on the horizon like a frieze. In my mind's eye I saw, as in a witch's ball, the figure of myself, spellbound" (52). Finally, in reading this scene, it is important not to lose sight of the fact that it was the young boy's choreography—a homoerotic dance performance—that opened emotive passages so that the participants could move towards the ecstatic epiphany that marks the after-dinner celebration.

Hassan el-Balbeissi

Running contrary to travel narrative orthodoxy, Flaubert does not closet his enthusiasm over the male dancers he observes in Cairo. As with Kuchuk Hanem, the experience becomes, in fact, the object of camaraderie in his correspondence with his close friend Louis Bouilhet (as we saw in chapter 3). However, even Flaubert, a writer eager to "play openly" during his travels, cannot resolve the profound ambivalence he feels over a male performer who overwhelms him before he meets Kuchuk Hanem. In January of 1850, he writes to Louis Bouilhet from Cairo describing the male dancers he has seen and identifying one of them as Hassan el-Balbeissi:

> As dancers, imagine two rascals, quite ugly, but charming in their corruption, in their obscene leerings and the effeminacy of their movements, dressed as women, their eyes painted with antimony.... The dancers advance and retreat, shaking the pelvis with a short convulsive movement. A quivering of the muscles is the only way to describe it; when the pelvis moves, the rest of the body is motionless; when the breast shakes, nothing else moves. In this manner they advance toward you, their arms extended, rattling brass castanets, and their faces, under the rouge and the sweat, remain more expressionless than a statue's. By that I mean they never smile. The effect is produced by the gravity of the face in contrast

86

*The Dance of
Extravagant
Pleasures:
Male
Performers
of the Orient
and the
Politics of
the Imperial
Gaze*

to the lascivious movements of the body. Sometimes they lie down flat on their backs, like a woman ready to be fucked, then rise up with a movement of the loins similar to that of a tree swinging back into place after the wind has stopped.... From time to time, during the dance, the impresario, or pimp, who brought them plays around them, kissing them on the belly, the arse, and the small of the back, and making obscene remarks in an effort to put additional spice into a thing that is already quite self-evident. (*Letters* 110-11)

Evidently, Flaubert finds this performance overwhelming and even comments that "I doubt whether we shall find the women as good as the men; the ugliness of the latter adds greatly to the thing as art" (111). The contradictions in Flaubert's description are a sign of his disorientation, as he finds himself teased into an uncertain space signified by the performance and also by the dancers' makeup and dress. Through contraries, he struggles to circumscribe the male dancers' performance but ultimately enunciates and reiterates his own ambivalence since the dance resists a written description in the viewer's imperial language. What Flaubert sees, evidently, is a compelling demon of the male sex luring him into realization of perverse sexual possibilities. In fact, with his behaviour during the performance, the impresario turns the already lascivious dance into a profane ritual that redirects Flaubert's masculine desire onto a transgressive course. In fact, this flirtation with Egyptian sodomy inspires a homoerotic exchange with his addressee, Louis Bouilhet, "and injects into Flaubert's correspondence and diaries a stream of homoerotic banter and speculation that becomes a source of titillation and eventually the spur to experimentation without radically disturbing the writer's heterosexual self-definition" (Boone 55). The insistence on Hassan's ugliness, in fact, seems a gesture to underscore the illicitness of this entire process of watching, an attempt to mask appeal with non-appeal. Ugliness, in other words, turns into a cherished aesthetic that is meant to trope the illicit desires that possess Flaubert.

In subsequent letters, however, Flaubert's sexual confidence gives way to a subliminal anxiety arising from his encounter with Near Eastern homosexuality and linked to his literary ambitions. According to Joseph Boone, "having traveled to Egypt in search of creative inspiration, Flaubert expresses his writerly potential in metaphors of heterosexual reproduction ('but—the real thing! To ejaculate, to beget the child!') and conversely expresses his despair at not having realized his literary goals in images of non-reproductive sexual play; he subtly figures the exotic others of sexual perversion as the great threat of erasure, the negation of artistic vitality or sap, when 'the lines don't come'" (55). Although ostensibly fascinating to Flaubert, Hassan el-Balbeissi's dancing is destabilizing, an effect that Flaubert hopes to amend with his torpid affair with Kuchuk Hanem, who fulfills the stereotype of the feminine Orient that is imagined as available and must be penetrated by Western superior intellect.

Flaubert's homosexual experiences are not detailed with the same intensity. Edward Said picks up on Flaubert's heterosexual narratives and elaborates on them theoretically. In such interpretations, the ghaziya's body has been read, correctly I think, as a trope for the earth that is ploughed and tilled. However, Hassan el-Balbeissi's body can be neither envisioned in similar images nor allowed the same possibilities by Flaubert—a disavowal that theorists such as Said have permitted by their silence on Hassan el-Balbeissi. Flaubert is the privileged khawadja (the white seigneur) who never transcends his gendered longing. He boasts of homosexual sex in the baths, but it is Kuchuk he hopes to subdue through scopic conquest and sexual possession.[11]

Nerval's Dancing "Girls"

My final paradigm involves an incident that Gerard de Nerval recounts as part of his Oriental adventures. A pleasant afternoon in the finest cafe in the fashionable area of Mousky provides the occasion for his first experience of Cairo's famous dancing "girls" in a public performance. In his travelogue, *The Women of Cairo; Scenes of Life in the Orient*, he relates the following:

> The dancing girls appeared in a cloud of dust and tobacco smoke.... As their heels beat upon the ground, with a tinkle of little bells and anklets, their raised arms quivered in harmony; their hips shook with a voluptuous movement; their form seemed bare under the muslin between the little jacket and the low loose girdle, like the ceston of Venus. They twirled around so quickly that it was hard to distinguish the features of these seductive creatures, whose fingers shook little cymbals, as large as castanets, as they gestured boldly to the primitive strains of flute and tambourine. Two of them seemed particularly beautiful; they held themselves proudly: their Arab eyes were brightened by kohl, their full yet delicate cheeks were lightly painted. (64)

Nerval's description is well within the familiar colonial schema of elaborate verbal depiction. Because this is a dancing scene, however, I read

The Dance of
Extravagant
Pleasures:
Male
Performers
of the Orient
and the
Politics of
the Imperial
Gaze

these details with an interest in deciphering the complex corporealization of the objects of his gaze. They incorporate elements which are familiar from other descriptions of both male and female Eastern performers: the striking and outlandish costumes, the makeup worn by the dancers, and their finger cymbals are ubiquitous features. Here their features are enhanced by an extra touch of eroticism that the "ceston of Venus" bestows. This item of their costume acquires multivalent significance as it registers the dance moves, thus enhancing the motion, but also as it embraces the hips acting in this capacity as a material manifestation of the gaze as it circles tightly but longingly, it would seem, the same part of the body.

In fact, Nerval's account of the khawals forms a particularly clear exemplar of the complex dynamics of makeup, costuming adornments, and finger cymbals as worn and played by Middle Eastern dancers. Because the analysis I suggest constructs dance itself as a narrative of sorts, I regard makeup and jewellery to be an indispensable component of this narrative. Along with physical movement and the sonic dimension that the finger cymbals reify, the metamorphosis of makeup and costume afford the passage that Nerval (and indeed any audience) is keen to witness. This narrative of metamorphosis is a central issue in discussions of Middle Eastern dance where, in the observer's gaze, the dancer's made-up eyes are such an arresting signifier. As the male dancers shift constantly before Nerval, their eyes *look* both transitively and intransitively, framed as they are by the black kohl.

The makeup around their eyes and on their face, the objects of self-adornment, and even the brass finger cymbals enhance the performativity of the body. Objects of adornment and embroidered costumes afford a physical metamorphosis essential for the body, both in its preparation for and through the duration of the dance. Moreover, they serve as markers of this potentiality in the viewer's gaze, while simultaneously setting up a semiotic system that invites the gaze yet guards the body in its creative and therefore vulnerable moments. To assist and illustrate my argument, I draw from the old Cypriot dialect where a term and its meanings evoke intriguing signs. The verb "kholiazo" derives from kohl and means, of course, to make oneself up but, oddly enough, it is also a word used in building and construction work. The same verb describes the process of filling up with grouting the gaps between slabs or tiles laid on a floor or against a wall. Therefore, "kholiazo" clearly implies placing something in-between in order to fill up space that would otherwise remain blank. The effect is one of embellishment but also strength since grouting also secures and keeps tiles or slabs in place. Perhaps it was this quality of makeup, functioning as an emboldening and in-between agent, that scandalized and irritated but also allured Europeans. It seemed to correct the vulnerability of nature by fortifying the performer with the drama of artifice. Thus, it denied the viewer straight access to the "nature" of the subject's face while also conjuring an image that was relentlessly seductive. (I use *straight* in its puritan sense, conscious also of its heterosexual connotations, and I use the word *nature* to imply both human character and physical look or physiognomy.) All the while, this artifice in the form of makeup and adornments fills gaps in performativity, strengthens it, and keeps the artistic body in a position whose condition is both distinguished and equivocated.

Indeed, adornment and maquillage merit an examination in the same terms as dance. They come alive on the dancing body in a fashion similar to a move. They practise a choreographed intervention on the natural body that affects not only the performance of the body's movement but also its sexuality. Their sheer presence, in other words, enacts the dance itself and subjugates the gaze just as kinesthesia does. Perhaps this is where the eroticism and exoticism associated with makeup become apparent and directly relevant. Makeup is erotic because it brings about a metamorphosis that follows auto-eroticism (as I comment earlier in my discussion of kohl in chapter 1). Further, "art" and artifice here may take on sexual connotations in that the artist ritually adorns herself, enhancing the performative potential of her body and thereby its sexualness.

Transformed, the dancing body transcends the rigidity of its physical form and acquires an altered dimension that excludes Nerval and his discriminations regarding gendered makeup customs. And during this entire ritual, the viewer is invited to the spectacle, which, in a sense, owes its existence to the viewer's gaze. Nevertheless, the dancer's masquerade denies the viewer the experience of the ritual. That is, ritual is for participants, not viewers. This is confirmed by bell hooks in her definition of ritual and spectacle in her critique of Jennie Livingston's film *Paris Is Burning*, a film whose black drag performances offer an intriguing parallel to Nerval's experience of the "effeminate" dancing boys:

> Ritual is that ceremonial act that carries with it meaning and significance beyond what appears, while spectacle functions primarily as entertaining dramatic display. Those of us who have grown up in a segregated black setting where we participated in diverse pageants and rituals know that those

90

The Dance of
Extravagant
Pleasures:
Male
Performers
of the Orient
and the
Politics of
the Imperial
Gaze

elements of a given ritual that are empowering and subversive may not be readily visible to an outsider looking in. Hence it is easy for white observers to depict black rituals as spectacle. (150)

I could not suggest that dancing was indeed "empowering and subversive" for the khawals in this particular scene (although I have certainly experienced dance in these terms; this is, in fact, why I dance). My point here follows bell hooks, who insists that a white (or in this case Western) gaze, watching a racialized "pageant" that it cannot decipher, translates it, instead, into mere spectacle. That is, the materialization of spectacle depends, to a certain extent, on the privilege of the viewer, although, as I argue, the boundaries of this privilege do not remain fixed but are contested by dance as ritual and as spectacle.

However, the ceremony that Nerval is hosting for us does not conclude here. He informs us that his enthusiastic participation in the scene is curtailed as soon as he becomes conscious that the dancers are not female but male: "But the third, I must admit, betrayed the less gentle sex by a week-old beard; and when I looked into the matter carefully, and, the dance being ended, could better make out the features of the other two, it did not take me long to discover that the dancing girls were, in point of fact, all males" (64). Perhaps predictably, since Nerval is addressing a mainstream, bourgeois audience, the fooled viewer immediately suspends his *pothos* and shifts the mechanisms of his gaze towards these deceitful performers.[12] They have embezzled his ethics, mocked his taboos, and made him complicit through his gaze in a lubricious spectacle: "I was ready to place upon their foreheads a few pieces of gold, in accordance with the purest traditions of the Levant.... But for men dressed up as women this ceremony may well be dispensed with, and a few paras thrown to them instead" (65). It is noteworthy how Nerval stages this spectacle for himself and for his reader. Although he excitedly details the performance of these dancers, he relates only in the title of this section, "The Khowals [sic]"—for those who know already that this is the Arabic for male dancers—that his "dancing girls" are, in fact, dancing boys. This play might lend itself to what we would term a "queer" reading in contemporary terms. He is enamoured of these boys only to be frustrated at the moment of gender recognition, yet he seems unwilling to protect his male readers from the same frustration by forewarning them. In this dissimulative restaging he has already communicated his erotic covetousness, so he could be expecting to incite it in his readers also. Along with the use of the term "queer," a further anachronism would be to call Nerval homophobic, although, according to Ramsay Burt's commentary on homosexuality and the male dancer, the term "homophobic" might well be appropriate here, since "Western society is and has for hundreds of years been profoundly homophobic" (29).[13] Nevertheless, nothing other than fascination with these alien, dancing bodies would urge Nerval to be as whimsical with his scenario and with his reader.

Later, he engages in the deprecation we are accustomed to reading in travel narratives where the immoral East is admonished for its depravity. He cleverly substitutes the wonder of artistic epiphany—those revelations, psychic and cognitive that a performance may induce in an audience—with the revelation of the dancers' sex and then proceeds to interpolate some imperial discourse that will further spoil the attraction of the ritual and denigrate the practice of male dancing:

> Seriously, there is something very peculiar about Egyptian morality. A few years ago, the dancing girls used to go freely about the city.... Now, they are only allowed to appear in private houses and banquets, and scrupulous people consider these dances by men with effeminate features and long hair, with bare arms, figures and necks, who parody so deplorably the half-veiled attractions of the dancing girls, more respectable. (65)

Even if his intention was to be sarcastic in this description of the dancing scene, he certainly is not convincing that these boys' quivering arms, voluptuous hips, and visible bare forms are deplorable parodies. Evidently, his pronouncements here do not attest to his depiction of the khawals. There is a tone of hostility in his refusal to transgress the moral boundaries of his culture whose morality he sees as too superior to compromise. There is something reminiscent of Charles Sonnini's hysteria in Nerval's expression of derision. Both men register reactions that foreclose the different kinds of contamination that Egypt, as a nation of the potent Orient, is capable of.

Finally, this scene from Nerval's narrative supports Anthony Shay's contention that male dancers were almost always discernible from females in the iconographic and narrative sources. Male dancers "did not specifically wear female garb, but rather special clothing and costumes suitable to show off their movements and to make them unique and attractive as dancers and entertainers" ("The Male Dancer" 19). In colonial travel narratives, however, the transformation afforded by makeup and jewellery, as well as henna and opulent, flamboyant, and dramatic costumes was feared and therefore criticized in women of the Orient. My contrapuntal readings of these travel narratives communicate

92

*The Dance of
Extravagant
Pleasures:
Male
Performers
of the Orient
and the
Politics of
the Imperial
Gaze*

the ways in which a dancer's makeup and personal adornment begin to appear threatening in their defiance of hegemony. In an effort to neutralize the effects of this transformation and the intense sexualization of the body that results from their adoption, male travellers and writers sought to explain them in terms of female "inconstancy" and waywardness. To observe such demonstrations in men, however, was too taxing on European sensibility.

Mousbah Baalbaki

As a conclusion to this chapter, I would like to relate the content of an article by Susan Sachs concerning a contemporary male dancer in Beirut. The article appeared in the *New York Times Beirut Journal* on 4 May 2000 and carried the unfortunate title "He's No Salomé, but It's Straight from the Heart." The dancer referred to, Mousbah Baalbaki, emerges from the article like a contemporary Hassan el-Balbeissi, gazing through "eyes rimmed with black powder." The reference to makeup is a necessary and, to my taste, a particularly appealing and significant part of the description, as in Nerval's description of the khawals. My purpose in discussing the article is partly to trace certain enduring patterns from the past to the present, although I do not wish to trap Mousbah, and myself, in a Romantic vision of the same dancing figure performing unaltered through time in a cliché template of the "timeless Orient." There is continuation in him, not in a Romantic Orientalist sense, but in the dynamics that have marked male performances through colonial and recently postcolonial times. The reporter finds him "sinuous and seductive … in a gauzy black caftan over a Bedouin-style white robe, [as] he undulated on stage with a faraway look in his eyes and a bodyguard close at hand." The writing adopts the traditional and, sadly, anticipated tone that ranges between sardonic and superior—an efficient and popular technique for relating information about something titillating, enticing, and "different." The same technique quells the anxiety that rises not just in the observing reporter, as is the case here, or the traveller but also in the reader. Hence the comments on the artistic components and "character" of the show: the melody of the old Arabic song sounds "lugubrious" and there is the assurance that "Mr. Baalbaki, who is 28, does not perform a transvestite show or a striptease. It is more like 'Saturday Night Fever' meets 'The Thousand and One Nights.'" These latter two productions are both Western constructs to varying degrees, which serves to leave the dancer unaccommodated and exiled between two worlds that he has had no agency in defining. Similarly, Lebanon itself is projected as a country that, "for all its worldly glitter" (that is, capitalist "development" and therefore general approval, familiarity, and comfort with the image—something reminiscent of the Eurovision Song Contest cosmopolitanism), still has "a generous streak of religious conservatism and criminalizes homosexuality." In other words, it remains "Oriental," which here implies stubbornly backward. Beirut itself is "a paradoxical town, with European designer boutiques interspersed with the sniper-shattered buildings from the fifteen-year civil war.... But Mr. Baalbaki's public gyrations seem a step beyond the pale even for Beirut" (Sachs).

It seems, however, that the journalist is not the only agent confining the male body's dance expression. Rather, in reiterating the paradox of Beirut, an "Oriental" city, the journalist is simply re-presenting the complexities of a postcolonial state of affairs since, in its modernity, Lebanese society itself displays values and morals that seem closer to those of Europe than traditional Arab society. Thus Mousbah's taboo performance invokes contemporary politics, national and international, and forms a most intriguing moment in postcolonial politics that is comparable to the Greek politics of Eastern dance (as I argue in detail in chapter 5). His body in motion becomes a crossroads where native tradition, colonialism, Lebanese class issues, and personal artistic ambition and adoration converge. "Every weekend," Mousbah claims, "I struggle with the audience." Indeed, the night Susan Sachs was at the "Amor y Libertad," she noticed men "squirm and concentrate resolutely on their drinks when Mr. Baalbaki took the stage."

Baalbaki's condemnation, however, comes from within the profession as well. Although he acknowledges the struggles that professional female dancers face in a culture that is generally harsh in its judgement of dancers, his support of them remains unreciprocated by his colleague Fifi Abdou, whom Sachs calls "the leading lady of Egyptian belly dancing." In a modest estimation of her contribution to the art form, Abdou "describes herself as the only living symbol of the art" (Sachs). Her charisma, prestige, and popularity are indisputable and they have made her one of the wealthiest Egyptian belly dancers (it is important to allude to her elevated class status). However, what have proven her most valuable contributions to the art were her "daring" interpretations of Oriental dance, her ability to perform a sexuality and an eroticism that, in the words of Cassandra Lorius, "outwit patriarchy" (287). I agree with Lorius's assessment that,

*The Dance of
Extravagant
Pleasures:
Male
Performers
of the Orient
and the
Politics of
the Imperial
Gaze*

when interpreting the dance, Fifi Abdou "makes use of play, a disjunc-
tive tactic that works against the potential closure of normative discourse" (287).[14] Despite her significant victories, however, Fifi Abdou is
intent on denying Mousbah, and every male dancer, the very ability to
perform this dance. She argues based on assumed biological properties of
the two sexes, as she explains in Susan Sach's article: "it's impossible for
a man to dance *real* belly dancing. The phrase itself describes the part from
the hips to the waist, and a man lacks the energy there that a woman has.
They can perform, but they can't belly-dance" (my emphasis). Seemingly
unconscious of the cultural weight her argument bears, Fifi Abdou—
ironically a native dancer herself who, apparently, continues to fight battles on the cultural field—crystallizes in her objection the very essence of
discomfort, anxiety, and allure felt by Western observers for male Oriental dancers. Even if the effort to "naturalize" the female performers
achieves some limited fulfillment (realized most strongly in the sexual
availability of these dancers' bodies), the effort to achieve the same with
men is simply impossible to fulfill politically in Western body discourse.
The male body has limitations, Fifi instructs us, and cannot perform the
"real" dance—with all the problematic denotations of the term "real."
The male dancer's invitation to experience an altered, othered dimension of reality and gendered space offers what is impossible to accept and
therefore denied at the body, the very source of its corporeal creation.

In a sense, the male dancer has remained resistant to familiariza-
tion, exacerbating the anxiety felt over the male dancing body. Thus,
when a dance instructor urges me, nervously and with some anxiety, not
to overdo my undulations or to render my moves with machismo (they
usually require sharper shoulder thrusts and less "eloquence and flair"
in the hands) she is, in effect, trying to unsettle my body's resistance to
normalized masculinity and hoping to reinstall something familiar, in this
case a conventional masculine character, in the spectacle of the male
dancer. At the same time the instructor is protecting herself and the audience. They stand on guard against the threatening opprobrium that would
assault gender propriety by suggesting the unspeakable.

If I can return to this chapter's opening paragraphs that outline certain events concerning the life of public dancers in Egypt in the 1830s, I
find it intriguing how these events have been constructed as historical
truth by modern dance researchers and dance enthusiasts. The information that, following Mohamed Ali's edict, there was heavier taxation to
compensate for lost revenue and that the dance scene became inundated

with dancing boys comes from Morroe Berger's article (30). Berger footnotes Lane as his source, yet Lane nowhere says that boys came along to substitute the girls in public performances. In fact, Lane's phobia regarding the khawals is such that he even denies they were a large population: "the number of these male performers," he insists, "is very small" (389). Regardless, Wendy Buonaventura reiterates that same information as Berger, presenting it as historical fact in *Serpent of the Nile* (68). These inferences and conclusions require further revision because despite being appealing in their historical tidiness, their character seems rather simplistic.

Islamic social rules, the narrative goes, prohibit women from public dancing; therefore men do it. The head of state decided to reform his society so he exiled the courtesans to Upper Egypt. Dancing boys came to prevail in their wake. These males were more salacious and obscene than the women. I outline these "facts" in order to point to the contradictory nature of the accounts we have been bequeathed. Also, this outline throws into relief a rather reductionist tendency towards the "Orient" itself: the notion that a few simple deductions drawn from a simple outline of events can explain away Eastern social and cultural phenomena and traditions. Meanwhile, even though the sources I have looked at hold that these events did in fact take place, they also refute them. Covel's and Schuyler's accounts indicate that male dancers belonged to a matured and highly valued tradition in the East. That they prevailed merely because female performance was interdicted by religious laws seems an unwarranted rationalization in the case of a successful and cherished cultural institution. Moreover, what lies in the imperative of explications such as Schuyler's (the boys dance because it is indecent for women to perform publicly) seems to be a need to excuse male presence in an artistic profession. Male performances were often seen as lewd and extremely improper but, as I have tried to show in this chapter, this response entails emotions that were a direct corollary of imperial status. Disgust is a form of self-policing—a means to arrest desire and catch the body before it assimilates the experience of dance with any amount of pleasure. Moreover, disgust is also the feeling we register when something that is internal and invisible and expected to remain so externalizes itself. The experience of dance is visceral and the emotion evoked by the gaze is disgust because the performing body gestures towards carnal alternatives whose very visual suggestion implicates the viewer. In the case of Middle Eastern dance, especially when performed by men or boys, viewers prefer to resist the acknowledgement of possibilities that the dancing body

96

The Dance of
Extravagant
Pleasures:
Male
Performers
of the Orient
and the
Politics of
the Imperial
Gaze

signifies. Such resistance, along with the willingness to represent and explicate Eastern cultural practices in uncomplicated terms, constitutes an act of violence against forms of kinesthetic, sexual, and gender embodiment that lie outside sanctioned norms.

The European gaze translated the experience of Eastern dance into a medium of aberrance and illicitness. In the Western imaginary, the dancer's body loomed threatening and enticing, mapping, in motion always, an intermediate zone, a threshold signifying liminality and indeterminacy, qualities often used to represent the East as a whole. Dancing women were a threat but at least their dancing body could be subjected to symbolic Western domination through sexual intercourse. Male dancers clothed in an Eastern form of drag posed an insurmountable challenge by occupying yet a further liminal space. Marjorie Garber articulates this threat in deconstructive terms: "If transvestism offers a critique of binary sex and gender distinctions, it is not because it simply makes such distinctions reversible but because it denaturalizes, destabilizes, and de-familiarizes sex and gender *signs*" (147). The "revelation" that the dancing girls were really boys—this revelation being the moment when Nerval actually deciphered the "sign"—is the moment when Nerval has to slip from the role of mere observer into that of the imperial moralist so he will not surrender to aberrance. Imperatively, his response puts him at variance with the Janissaries, the hot-blooded sultan's soldiers, as Eastern spectators of a similar spectacle. In direct defiance of Eastern practices, he wants to throw a few *paras* to the dancers, because by throwing he will not have to take another look at them; looking could make voyeuristic indulgence in Oriental perversion a very real possibility. I should point out that this perversion may effect a two-way manifestation: the dancing boys will also look at Nerval and their gaze will penetrate his masculinity. Perhaps their "unnaturalness" signals to him the arbitrariness of his own gender and sexuality.

The encounters with male dancers that I have examined provide some unique manifestations of the necessarily sexual performance of the look that informs both the practice and the concept of the gaze. The Orient had to become crystallized in the image of the fecund, sexually insatiable woman, even though there existed significant opportunity for Western travellers to restructure this image of the Orient. Yet, to acknowledge the male dancer as an emblem would also acknowledge him as a "designated repository of sexuality" (Shay, "The Male Dancer" 20) in which the Western male tourist was investing his desire. To replace the ghawazee with the khawals, çengi, koçek, or batchas would be re-presenting a mas-culinized West that penetrates a male Orient—nothing less than an act of sodomy. Besides, much of the pleasure derived from this imaginary penetration predicated itself upon the constructed image of the Orient as a fecund, "feminized space" (McClintock 26). This image afforded a perverse and abstract but very crucial and gratifying notion of fertiliza-tion. Such was the satisfaction Flaubert needed to delude himself with. Sexual encounters with Hassan el-Balbeissi, or any other male sex part-ner, could not have provided the same possibility. The liminal space these male dancers occupied, a space in between genders, may have tantalized, titillated, or appalled the Western bourgeois traveller, but it never inspired an openly expressed feeling of comfort. Policed by their culture's taboos, these travellers needed a firm foothold at either the masculine or femi-nine threshold, even when they relished sexual experiences with cross-dressed performers.

The dancers were not isolated in inciting curiosity and hate, attrac-tion, and repulsion. The East as a whole generated the same emotional effects. The white European's emotions regarding the spectacle of dance—fear, shock, disgust—set in motion those mechanisms that reinstate in the traveller's gaze the superiority of European culture and its elite embod-iment. The Middle Eastern male dancer, with the made-up eyes and the "lascivious" movements, posed—indeed, continues to pose—a particu-lar threat that had to be contested and its injurious effects exorcised. However, the male dancer would not be entirely censored from the nar-ratives since his form, constantly shifting in the condition of dance, is necessary in the Empire's constant redefining of itself against the Orien-tal Other. Out of this incessant choreography and the Empire's cease-less revisions of its predicaments, rose the body of Salomé. She became the royal figure whose legendary dance and ignominious request acquired a particularly valuable currency in the latter half of the nineteenth cen-tury, precisely because her image qualified as at once appalling and enchanting, androgynous and feminine, desiring and destructive.

4 / Dancing Decadence
Semiotics of Dance and the Phantasm of Salomé

Between her fingers her noisy castanets tinkled and rang unceasingly. *"Cawadja*, what do you think of Kuchuk Hanem now?" she cried, as she writhed her hips. She held out her two long arms, black and glistening, shaking them from shoulder to wrist with an imperceptible quivering, moving them apart with soft and quick motions like those of the wings of a hovering eagle. Sometimes she bent completely over backwards, supporting herself on her hands in the position of the dancing Salomé over the left portal of the Rouen cathedral.

Maxime du Camp, "Le Nil, Egypte et Nubie"

(Steegmuller, *Flaubert in Egypt*)

In this chapter, I will examine ways in which Salomé's dance and its associated decapitation of a Christian saint relate to colonial dynamics. One of the fundamental premises of my argument is that while watching dance, the gaze cannot remain passive or complacent in its assumed superiority. In scopic indulgence, the eye consumes the dancer and the dance, ingests the spectacle, and assimilates it in a manner that interrogates any notions of purity in an imperial subject's sovereign constitution. In fact, the seduction of the dance is capable of causing disruption in the Empire through a fracture within the imperial body itself, hence the vehement responses to the male dancers that I have discussed. Gerard de Nerval does not wish to sustain his gaze on the khawals because the scopic exchange at that particular instant feminizes his masculine and heterosexual subjectivity. And, even more threatening, when the khawals turn their gaze upon him, their scopic gesture permeates and dis-

 Notes to chapter 4 are on page 210.

*Dancing
Decadence:
Semiotics
of Dance
and the
Phantasm of
Salmomé*

solves (even momentarily) his manly integrity. However, not all Europeans share the same kind of investment in such masculinity. What Nerval avoids with apparent annoyance while he is on tour, Oscar Wilde's *Salomé* attempts to stage in the heart of the Metropolis. The vitality of an "exotic" dance performance can realize a metamorphosis that allows for possibilities indispensable to the decadent imagination. I wish to link the textual reading of Wilde's play and his own sexual politics as they configure exotic and domestic politics of imperialism and Middle Eastern dance. Because Wilde's Salomé is scandalous, I will also stipulate a certain occasional identification of Salomé with Wilde in the effort to foreground Victorian sexual politics and their link to colonialism. "Scandal," Smaro Kamboureli posits, "is a sign of excess and transgression, but also of violation and indignity" (ix). The decadent Salomé is an archetypal and notorious "scandalous body" (in identifying her as such, I wish to also place her within Kamboureli's focus on diasporic bodies because Salomé qualifies, in a number of ways, as a diasporic body). In Wilde's treatment she is precisely "a sign of excess and transgression," but also of "violation and indignity"—an allusion to the court injunction against Wilde's homosexual "extravagances."

In keeping with the larger endeavour, I will attempt to locate and interrogate dance's challenging transformation within the schema of imperial interpretations of Middle Eastern dance as excessive movement that disrupts the boundaries of gender definition. My discussion foregrounds the symbolist thematics of Salomé and her decadent insurrection, examined within the framework of empire. The decadent writer's genius relies for its progress on the exposition of an exoticism and an eroticism that are made possible through kinesthetic movement. "The exotic and the erotic ideals go hand in hand," Mario Praz indicates; "the love of the exotic is usually an imaginative projection of a sexual desire" (197). Edward Said echoes Praz's equation but exposes the tensions implicit in such a formula: "Why the Orient seems still to suggest not only fecundity but sexual promise (and threat), untiring sensuality, unlimited desire, deep generative energies, is something on which one could speculate" (188). However, what particularly interests me is how this equation of exoticism and eroticism modifies itself before Oriental dance. Indeed, much of the unceasing, decadent circulation of the exotic-turned-erotic draws the strength of its cultural impact from the trope of dance in travel narratives, while the trope itself turns on the imperial jurisdiction over sexuality, race, and gender. In fact, the dancers whom Flaubert and others observed and constructed narratively inspired a literary output that was decidedly shaped by exotic movement and sexualness. However, Wilde's *Salomé* is one of the few texts that thematize lucidly the intricate economies of scopophilia, transformation, and, of course, dance movement, although gazing itself, in the play, also possesses the energy of a choreography; looking sets both the plot and itself into a dance. Salomé, her dance, and its consequence, are never in want of reference. Yet even though she has received a great deal of attention, she has not often been adequately linked to the ways in which colonial politics affected the rediscovery and recirculation of Salomé as an aesthetic figure, or to Wilde's exceptional treatment of her.

Roughly sketched, the discussion will move in three sections, each one responding to related questions. First, I will briefly examine the extent to which travel narratives and their imperial inscription affected decadent Salomania. I will, therefore, assess the importance and influence of representations of Middle Eastern dancers—the "native Salomés"—in travel narratives and their ideological sublimation into the foreboding Salomé of the *fin de siècle*. This brief examination will foreground certain racial dynamics that attended this biblical figure's decadent constructions. Second, what sort of impact did this legacy of the dancing female exotic have on Wilde's influential recreation of Salomé? It is important to consider what he retained and what he discarded in the process of amalgamating sexual and Orientalist politics in a performance (theatrical and personal) that ultimately dismantled his status as father, man of letters, and public figure, and brought about his total ruin. Tangential to Wilde's trial are other prosecutions of scandalous Salomés whose performativity revolves around the same configuration of sexuality, dance, and nationality. These prosecutions will comprise my third area of interest. Here I aim to assess the Orientalism of Salomé's various performances by responding to questions regarding their "authenticity." In other words, how "authentic" was her performance and how did such quality affect the constant negotiation of sexuality, race, and Empire?

Salomé as a Native Figure

The native images that the colonial gaze collected and represented to itself were transported back to the Metropolis in a recoded form. These images carried more than the value of mere mementos from the trip and they were more than innocent reminders of native emotional or expres-

102

Dancing
Decadence:
Semiotics
of Dance
and the
Phantasm of
Salmomé

sive practices. Through journal records, retelling, and remembering, these images were transformed into imaginary artefacts from the peripheral culture that, upon their return, the travellers declared at an excited cultural customs office of sorts—the moment of declaration often resembling a greedy male rite. Images of native dancers were particularly prized items in this process. In the final part of chapter 2, we saw the significance of Azizeh's dancing for Flaubert in her humble hut. Maxime du Camp, Flaubert's travelling companion, provides a more detailed portrayal of Azizeh and her performance. Here I provide the lengthy passage, part of which served as an epigraph to this chapter:

> She is elegant and almost awesome, with her black skin, like bronze in its nuances of green and copper; her crinkly hair, full of gold piastres, is barely covered by a yellow kerchief dotted with blue flowers: her markedly slitted eyes seem like silver globes inset with black diamonds, and they are veiled and languid like those of an amorous cat. Her white, even teeth glitter from behind the thin lips of her mouth; a long necklace of sequins hangs down to her belly, which is circled by a girdle of glass beads that I can see through the diaphanous folds of her clothing ... Between her fingers her noisy castanets tinkled and rang unceasingly. She held out her two long arms, black and glistening, shaking them from shoulder to wrist with an imperceptible quivering, moving them apart with soft and quick motions like those of the wings of a hovering eagle. Sometimes she bent completely over backwards, supporting herself on her hands in the position of the dancing Salomé over the left portal of the Rouen cathedral. (Steegmuller, *Flaubert in Egypt* 154-55)

What this description projects is, primarily, Maxime du Camp's effort to manage Azizeh's challenge, a way to access and capture her performance. Although the brief translation of the dance moves is intriguing (indeed, the suggestion of shoulder shimmies and back bends would be particularly appealing to anyone who is familiar with this dance vocabulary), the dancer herself appears somewhat grotesque and only semihuman. Her markedly "slitted eyes" transcend human form; they are more like jewels and no sooner are they depicted as lifeless precious stones than they are "veiled and languid" and, therefore, reminiscent of feline eyes. Du Camp's distortion of Azizeh's gaze is deliberate so that scopic control will rest entirely with his authority. Azizeh has no vision.

Moreover, the constantly shifting metaphors convey the evanescence of the dance itself and the impossibility of its visual "capture." Maxime du Camp deploys these shifting metaphors to transit through a racial—

and racist—definition of Azizeh that does not fix itself onto any particular racist construct familiar from anthropological or ethnographic discourses. His colonial desire—his intent to "know" her—conjures a series
of mixed metaphors that make whoever Azizeh is vanish even further in
his linguistic depiction. She is an amorous cat and a hovering eagle, languid, yet quivering with energy. The description of Azizeh and her dance
evokes images that affected the decadent movement profoundly. Baudelaire, for instance, relied on figures of the racialized female Other, the
cat, and dance extensively. (Stathis Gourgouris's comment that "Baudelaire is a genius insofar as he comes to monopolize the terms of 'Paris as
the capital of the nineteenth century'" (204) is quite astute and fitting.)
Along with all the images, Azizeh's dancing reminds du Camp of Salomé,
conceived in his description as an archetypal sign brimming with meanings.

   Although aligned with hieratic texts, Salomé's notorious and eternally mysterious "dance" has far-reaching psychological implications that
connect to an experience of the periphery as the site of formidable, mor-
bid, yet fascinating promises. The significance of her monumental performance and its consequence, the beheading of John the Baptist, saw
several re-enactments, ranging from the subtle to the obvious, in colonial travels. For example, while in Algiers in 1899, André Gide, who
Elaine Showalter informs us may have helped Wilde in writing *Salomé*
(149), echoes the same discourse of fear and fascination in a mystical
evocation that the dancers inspire:

> Here, between the stolid pillars of the hall, women are dancing, heavy
> and tall, not so much lovely as alien, and adorned to excess. They move
> slowly. The pleasure they sell is a solemn one, secret and powerful as
> death. Near the café, on a courtyard filled with moonlight or with shad-
> ows, each has her door ajar. Their beds are low—you lie down on them as
> in a grave. Pensive Arabs watch the dancers braid their steps to a music
> continuous as the sound of running water. A man serves coffee in a tiny
> cup—so tiny you might think you were drinking oblivion. (4-5)

The stygian gloom in Gide's narrative is a circulating motif in the exotic
travel experience. As Showalter posits, "the veiled woman, who is dangerous to look upon, also signifies the quest for the mystery of origins, the
truths of birth and death" (145). Although Gide's comment concerns
the "pleasure" these women sell, most likely alluding to their profession
as prostitutes, his point of reference here is not the hedonistic fulfillment
of sexual consummation, but a voyeuristic indulgence in the mysterious

104

*Dancing
Decadence:
Semiotics
of Dance
and the
Phantasm of
Salmomé*

erotics of death. Moreover, strongly pertinent are Azizeh's gold piastres, glass beads, and necklace of sequins, and, generally, the dancer's excessive adornment. This recurring and obsessive motif in the travel descriptions calls upon the veil as the mysterious artifact that is so often associated, somewhat vaguely, with an arcane Orient. Ornamentation and makeup, like the veil, contribute invaluably to the signification process of the exotic subject. Jewels and veils melt and mix at that magical point where scopic, fetishistic, and, ultimately, sexual rays of imperial desire converge. I see, therefore, Showalter's comment about the veiled woman as applicable to the adorned female Other as well. In both, the insignia function as formidable incarnations of life's aporias, those open spaces filled, paradoxically, with absent understandings of the mysteries of love, desire, and death.

In Flaubert, the dancers' mortal threat derives from a more direct biblical source than Gide's and is activated by a particular dance move. For example, head slides are a rhythmic movement of the head to both sides, a popular characteristic of dance traditions from several regions of the East. Flaubert finds this move to be a formidable act. Azizeh begins: "her neck slides back and forth on her vertebrae, and more often sideways, as though her head were going to fall off; terrifying effect of decapitation" (Steegmuller, *Flaubert in Egypt* 121). That this move was quite popular in the mid-nineteenth century becomes apparent in Flaubert's comment, "all the women have that movement of the head sliding on the vertebrae that so *astonished* us the first time" (my emphasis, 153). The psychoanalytic implications are fairly direct. The combination of fear and decapitation evoke the myth of Medusa, whose unshielded gaze literally astonished male subjectivity:

> According to Freud, the decapitated head of Medusa with its snaky looks is a "genitalized head," an upward displacement of the sexual organs, so that the mouth stands for the *vagina dentata*, and the snakes for pubic hair. For men to unveil the Medusa is to confront the dread of looking at the female sexual organs: "to decapitate: to castrate. The terror of Medusa is thus a terror of castration that is linked to the sight of something." (Showalter 145)

Certainly, the sight of Azizeh's "head slides" horrifies Flaubert, whose fear is displaced. Azizeh's head will become—perhaps it is already—the decapitated Medusa. Flaubert's terror presumably originates from the fear of castration, which symbolically translates into the erasure of his masculine subjectivity. Paradoxically, in this threat might lie the urgency for Flaubert's sexual consummation with the dancer after the performance. Performing "sex" (in both its meanings of gender and intercourse) becomes a means to mitigate this threat of female sexuality.

As if to augment the effect of decapitation, the dancer's expression often blocks or refracts the gaze, seemingly to refuse it entry or possession of the dance. Azizeh's face is "always expressionless" (Steegmuller, *Flaubert in Egypt* 122). Hassan el-Balbeissi and the unnamed male dancer performing with him similarly display the "expressionlessness of their faces under the streaks of rouge and sweat." Flaubert believes that "the effect comes form the gravity of the face contrasted with the lascivious movements of the body" (*Flaubert in Egypt* 70). Commenting on this aspect of the description, Andrea Deagon suggests that it signifies a projection of Flaubert's own conflicting needs and desires onto the Oriental Other:

> Regardless of cultural differences, Flaubert certainly imbued this expressionlessness with a meaning that attributed to the women of the Orient, and its male and female dancers, an issue that was deeply characteristic of his own nature: the split between sensual experience and true pleasure, between sexuality and emotional tenderness. Significantly, he does not focus on the idea of expressionlessness in his description of Kuchuk Hanem, with whom he apparently felt or longed to feel some real connection. ("Image of the Eastern Dancer" 14)

Expressionlessness could, therefore, be the manifestation of Flaubert's own conflicts. Furthermore, this formidable blankness of expression, that in Flaubert's eyes seems to signify a lack, serves to apprehend the viewer's gaze and by extension annihilate his hypostasis. This erasure partakes in the perpetuation of Salomé's construction as a ruthless and insatiable man-killer, while her dance functions as passage through which her insidious plot sees its gory realization. This whole scenario is enacted in the New Testament episode of John the Baptist's beheading.

Beyond this religiously inspired phobia, the sliding head movements along with the expressionless dancer's gaze generate the European gaze's predicament. The threat of castration, although isolating the viewer from the exotic realm whose reign he desires, also holds, paradoxically, a promising, albeit perverse, transformation that will flow from his defunct identity. Deagon's observations are astute when she points out how Kuchuk is never described as "expressionless." Yet, Flaubert had intimations of perilous misadventures even with the dancer who inspired him with the possibility of profound connections. Sleeping with Kuchuk and dozing off

106

Dancing
Decadence:
Semiotics
of Dance
and the
Phantasm of
Salmomé

with his fingers passed through her necklace, the image he conjures is again one of decapitation: "I thought of Judith and Holofernes sleeping together" (Steegmuller, *Flaubert in Egypt* 118). Judith is yet another biblical figure who seduced the Assyrian general Holofernes with her beauty, made him drunk, and beheaded him in his sleep (Tsianikas 62). By this murder she saved her country and herself from capture and enslavement. The motif that carries on into the Salomé legend is that the seduced male personalities are, in both Flaubert's experience and in religious lore, significant public figures with a great deal of influence—a theme that is particularly appealing to the khawadja, the white seigneur, whose self-image relies for its grandiosity on sensing his own elevated status. Significantly, the configuration of class and Western privilege replicates itself further in the biblical dancer of death. Salomé is also a princess who performs privately, for a select audience of privileged noblemen who stand in marked opposition to the deprived rabble who observe John the Baptist's preachings with their childlike rapture (Garelick 131).

The Legacy of the "Daughter of Sodom"

The original story of Salomé derives from the New Testament, namely the gospels of Matthew and Mark. Neither source, however, names Salomé as the perpetrator of the crime against St. John the Baptist; in fact, neither gospel names Salomé at all. In both texts, Salomé's mother, Herodias, seems to be the instigator, since she instructs her young daughter what to request following her performance. The Herodias of Matthew's version is particularly heinous, since she tutors her daughter before the performance on what to demand as reward, a premeditation that Flaubert reproduces and develops in his story "Herodias." "As we see," Sylvia Ellis writes, "the Bible portrays Salomé as less of a temptress than as a docile girl, and the responsibility for John's death lies firmly with Herodias. But it is the figure of Salomé, the dancer, which took on dimensions of immorality as time went by, until she is discovered as *femme fatale* of the Decadence amid trappings that become frankly barbaric and culminate in the grotesque" (14). Indeed, because of the dearth of detail in its biblical source, Salomé's legend has provided a perfectly empty slate to be carved with elaborate imperial motifs. The unnamed dancer and her unnarrated dance fledge into the metacolonial trope of a salacious and foreboding performance of racialized exotic femininity in the Western imaginary.

Salomé raises the spectre of Eastern female sexuality at a time when, as I discussed in chapter 2, the panoramic gaze interpreted the landscape of the Middle East in biblical terms. Helen Zagona scans the legend's chronicles and locates a resurgence in the late nineteenth century:

> Giving the legend's history a sweeping glance, we note that in its twenty-one-hundred-year course it has hit three peaks of interest: the first, in the period of Roman decadence; the second, in the Middle Ages; and the third in the post-romantic era, notably in France where the development of that frame of mind which eventually branded itself "décadent" was to provide the ideal esthetic climate for our subject. (22)

Significantly, and perhaps not coincidentally, this post-Romantic era that Zagona refers to is also the epoch of sexual and imperial anxieties. It was, therefore, the perfect climate for Salomé to dance her entrance as, in Garber's words, "a piece of domesticated exotica that confirms Western prejudices about the 'Orient' and about 'women' because it is produced by those prejudices, is in fact an exercise in cultural tautology" (340). Indeed, the myth of Salomé stirs "cultural and sexual fantasy" with a combination of themes such as "parents and a wilful child; incestuous desire; taboo" (Garber 340). Garber's breakdown of the elements tends to divest the legend of its mystic aura, which manipulates the legend's appeal quite effectively. Salomé gyrates through the *fin de siècle* wrapped in veils of anxiety, mystery, macabre horror, and above all, desire. She becomes the avatar of dance itself as conceived by decadent aestheticism: foreboding, alluring, fearful, irresistible, and full of possibility. And she emerges with airs of universality about her, arching her dancing body to bridge Orient and Occident, past and present.

In Wilde's drama, Salomé suggests continuity between the Roman, Judaic, and Christian religions and his own religion of art and sensuality. Coming from such a formidable configuration, it is no surprise that Salomé arrived at Wilde's play on transit from a variety of artistic conditions, painting and poetry being just two of these. Wilde inherited an extensive legacy of Salomé-inspired works since a large number of artists in the second half of the nineteenth century, especially French, were lovesick over the daughter of Herodias. In certain works, Salomé emerged as a potent and powerful feminine embodiment of male phobia and misogyny, while other creations wanted her to embody an erotic, sensual Orientalist vision. While offering a fresh interpretation of the biblical theme, Wilde's play acknowledges this variety of attitudes and artistic demands made of Salomé. "Heine is not the only master recalled in Salomé," Helen

Dancing
Decadence:
Semiotics
of Dance
and the
Phantasm of
Salmomé

Zagona points out; "all of Wilde's predecessors are in some manner represented therein: Mallarmé, Huysmans, Laforgue, and, above all, Flaubert" (121). What critics do not often dwell upon is that all these exponents of decadence were, like Baudelaire, geniuses because their production came to rest at the epicentre of French imperialism. Wilde's fantasy, however, although reliant on the canonical imperial matrix of responses, also designates a point of departure from that canon.

The effeminate garb and feminine performance of the khawals and the adroit Azizeh converge in Oscar Wilde's dancer. Garber argues that both in the biblical version and in its colonial adaptation, the myth incorporates a refusal to acknowledge transvestism as a destabilizing and defining agent:

> For the binary myth of Salomé—the male gazer (Herod), the female object of the gaze (Salomé); the Western male subject as spectator (Flaubert, Huysmans, Moreau, Wilde himself) and the exotic, feminized Eastern Other—this myth, a founding fable of Orientalism, is a spectacular disavowal. What it refuses to confront, what it declines to look at and acknowledge, is the disruptive element that intervenes, the scandal of transvestism. (339-40)

Although I agree with Garber, I also feel that Salomé's scope is wider than "the scandal of transvestism." The political schema that Salomé gave rise to in relation to Empire is endowed with certain complications. For example, Anne McClintock, while she finds Garber's work very useful, questions the scope of Garber's theory on cross-dressers as the transgressive embodiment of ambiguity. McClintock worries that "by universalizing all cross-dressers as transgressive ('the figure that disrupts') and by inscribing all fetishes as originating in the Lacanian castration scene ('the phallus is the fetish, the fetish is the phallus'), Garber does not do theoretical justice to the rich diversity of cultural cross-dressers and historical fetishes that she herself reveals" (67). In other words, Salomé's figure, as Andrea Deagon suggests, "became a significant trope in art, literature and aesthetic dance … reinterpreted to address complex issues of gender, power, sexuality, art, and foreignness" ("Dance of the Seven Veils" 2). Salomé's decadent cult was invigorated by the immediate experience of Middle Eastern dance and its narrativist construction in Western Europe and North America, and competed recklessly with colonial concerns. In the desire and derision that she invoked, Herodias's daughter became the trope of the archetypal dancing figure threatening to disrupt the imperial sexual order, a disruption that was of absolute necessity to the Empire.

Dance in Wilde's play does not exhaust the narrative and is not in turn exhausted by it. Movement is not ostentatious but subtle, while choreography as structured kinetic composition is absent. When the portentous moment approaches, the stage directions simply read, "Salomé dances the dance of the Seven Veils." Among the array of critics who have focused on the issue of dance (or, more appropriately, the absence thereof) is Amy Koritz. In *Gendering Bodies/Performing Art*, Koritz suggests that "Wilde again undercuts the polarization of the body and the soul, for the textual absence of the dance in effect spiritualizes the most purely physical moment of the play, just as the moment of the kiss is spiritualized by its invisibility" (82). In Koritz's reading, Salomé has to be put to death at the end of the play because she has sought to unify the exotic being (implying a fixity in her sensuality and eroticism) with the mystic (meaning transcendental and eternal), without relinquishing the place of her body (77-80). I can see how, in such an interpretation, dance may indeed make sense as a union of the body and the soul. "Body and soul" discourse, however, often seems concerned with a "union" that, although suggesting equal participation, inevitably relegates the physicality of the body to an inferior status. It is certainly worthy of more, since the body is the site where culture marks its control, history marks its passage, and where dance enacts its compliant resistance. Regarding it as mere conduit for the spirit places the body in an ascetic content that should rather be an obsolete idea. I am not suggesting that Koritz goes this far. In fact, she attributes the poor reception of the play and its condemnation to a social need "both to evade and to confirm the power and the threat of the exotic woman" (75). Engaging in a similar social critique, Elaine Showalter posits that the intricate gender blurring in Beardsley's illustrations of the play has gone unnoticed because of an obstinacy, even on the part of critics, to read such signs: "That so many critics have been blind to the meaning of the illustrations shows how cultural unwillingness to look at what is disturbing prevents us from seeing" (152). Such protestation against critics' ignorance of Beardsley's semiotics is an issue parallel with dance. Beardsley's drawings are like still dancing poses from the play: dance is ubiquitous, but its energy relies on our gaze to initiate its emanations.

I will return to the ubiquity of dance and its interaction with the audience once I revisit and elaborate further on another ubiquitous signifier: the veil. Andrea Deagon proposes that Wilde had clear intentions in naming it "the dance of the Seven Veils":

Dancing
Decadence:
Semiotics
of Dance
and the
Phantasm of
Salmomé

Wilde influentially defined the motion of Salomé's dance as unveiling, and clearly a woman unveiling was no simple thing, especially since the *modus operandi* of his play was shockingly to interweave passionate sexual desire with sacred texts. Neither Wilde nor the well-read among his audience could have been unaware of the common associations of veiling with initiation, and of sevens with sacred and mystical traditions: the seven seals of Revelations, the seven deadly sins, the seven sages, the seven stages of Mithraic initiation, the seven planets, etc. By combining the standard mystical number, the multivalent veil, and the revelation of the female body, in a context of a passionate conflict between a virgin's unbridled love and an ascetic's self-involved purity, Wilde knotted together ideas whose conflicts provided fruitful results in both controversy and performed interpretations. ("Dance of the Seven Veils" 3)

The mystical exaltation that Deagon suggests finds an artful accomplice in the veil. "It suggests the possibility of access to another sphere, another sexuality, another self," as Showalter indicates (148), and thus the veil becomes an indispensable, dramatic agent in the "shared mimetic process" (Garelick 135). Wilde sought to stage a *Salomé* whose choreography extracts from Middle Eastern dance a certain "mystique" that is imperative in catalyzing a transformation in which the male body invites this threatening fracture, ultimately with the intention of attaining a gender-transgressive identity—a feminization of sorts. Veiling as initiation, in Deagon's words, and the multilayered signification of the number seven, tinge the play's purpose with a certain flair that Rhonda Garelick quite aptly calls "camp" (her entire chapter is titled "Camp Salomé" 128-53). This transformation affords a welcome transcendence of masculine boundaries, an experience of a subjectivity that qualifies as excessive, taboo, and therefore scandalous in the Empire's material terms and spiritual pretensions.

Returning to Beardsley's illustrations to observe them in relation to the veil, I want to note Elaine Showalter's suggestions regarding veiling and sexual semiotics. Salomé's dance is potent because it gestures towards a potential breakdown of gender axioms, a formidable threat but also a captivating prospect. Such gender axioms are played out in Beardsley's set. His designs assume a role of stage management and direct Salomé's dance performance through their depictions. Showalter maintains that:

> Beardsley's drawings bring out all too powerfully the secret or unspeakable subtext of the play, especially its homoerotic and blasphemous elements. In the edition he presented to Beardsley, Wilde wrote: "For the only

artist who, besides myself, knows what the dance of the seven veils is and can see that invisible dance." The dance Beardsley sees is the dance of gender, the delicacy and permeability of the veil separating masculine from feminine, licit from illicit desire. (152)

Showalter concludes that Beardsley's illustrations support a "conflation of Wilde and Salomé, of female corrosive desire and male homosexual love, bring[ing] to the surface the play's buried and coded messages." (This is quite an accomplishment for Beardsley considering his lack of admiration for the play and his "cordial dislike" [Ross 17] of Wilde.)

The ritualistic inferences that Deagon outlines in relation to the veil, along with Beardsley's depictions and the play's language, are all forms of dance. Albeit without the formality of a choreographed presence, dance is embodied by this variety of agents, including the incantatory quality of the dialogue and, strangely, even the act of gazing itself:

The Young Syrian: How beautiful is the Princess Salomé to-night!

The Page of Herodias: Look at the moon. How strange the moon seems! She is like a woman rising form a tomb. She is like a dead woman. One might fancy she was looking for dead things.

The Young Syrian: She has a strange look. She is like a little princess who wears a yellow veil, and whose feet are of silver. She is like a princess who has little white doves for feet. One might fancy she was dancing.

The Page of Herodias: She is like a woman who is dead. She moves very slowly. (19)

The play's intense and lyrical tone derives from the "Song of Songs," a biblical passage whose sensuous references render it an exceptional moment in the original sacred text. But in the Wildean version, the "Song of Songs" is orchestrated *and* choreographed by the play's language. Here, motion is subtle and unconventional and so is the desired instrumentation by giant braziers of perfume that were intended to take the place of an orchestra (Showalter 150). A different scent was supposed to introduce each new emotion, a theatrical technique that, apart from being sensational, demolishes the boundary between audience and stage. The emotions would acquire an almost palpable manifestation that the audience can perceive with its senses. Garelick calls the result (which never materialized, unfortunately) "a synesthetic spectacle of startling effects":

In his imagination, however, the wafting clouds of perfume would replace the stage curtain, creating partial, diaphanous veils for the drama. His

*Dancing
Decadence:
Semiotics
of Dance
and the
Phantasm of
Salmomé*

conception of the theatrical space as both perfumed and veiled recalls, in these respects, the classically decadent conception of the Oriental dancing girl. Flaubert's Salammbô, for example, wore earrings made from perforated vials of scented oils, which slowly dripped their perfume over her body throughout the day. Wilde's braziers would treat as a dancing princess not only the entire stage, which would be drenched in perfume, but the audience as well, for its members would be equally scented, even after leaving the theater. (148)

Fire regulations did not permit the decadent extravagance that Wilde envisioned for his play. Nevertheless, we can decipher Wilde's purposes, as Garelick does quite astutely in her analysis. His ideas for the performance had multifarious purposes: audience seduction, the reification of an Orientalist vision, and a lasting scented effect that revolutionizes the perception of spectacle by distending the experience which will have touched the audience, both literally and figuratively.

The scented and colourful kinesthesis would be augmented by a constant and rigorous circulation of gazing, and dialogue against the background of a sacred tradition and Orientalist sensory appeal. All these diverse components sublimate the dance and transform it into a site of allurement and beguiling apprehensions. The poet himself invokes the seductive rhythm that resonates through all angles of the viewer, playwright, and dancer triangle. Desire circulates over all the images and mixed metaphors, reluctant to settle on a single object. As Garelick points out, Wilde's intervention in the Salomé legend lies in the way he melds into the entire play, characters included, what were hitherto exclusive characteristics of Salomé and her dance. To clarify her point, Garelick provides a brief synopsis of the decadent aesthetic of the femme-artiste, who provides the material that inspires the male artist to produce, and explains how Wilde, with *Salomé* in particular, intervened in the traditions that he had been bequeathed:

In this literature, the dancer and her dance stand for pure mimesis, and the creative process itself. The artist relies on this nonverbal writing for inspiration; he adds his words to the blank, gestural poem provided by the woman. Wilde's *Salomé* shatters this relationship; the dancer and the spectator lose their privileged places. Here, all the play's characters—not just two—act out a single, shared mimetic process, their words echoing with an eerie repetitiveness. It almost ceases to matter who is speaking, since the dialogue seems to live an independent life, detached from speakers' individual motives or psychology. (135)

Garelick's suggestion is valuable since, in her reading, Wilde's play instigates a new signification process in performance. *Salomé* can be read as a seminal text that reinvents the concepts of male inspiration and the possibilities of the dancer, the dance, and the audience. The incantatory quality of the dialogue is a technique that blurs the sharp contours expected to distinguish the characters and their different roles. Instead, as Garelick suggests, these distinctions dissolve into the text and, during performance, reach into the audience itself, which becomes implicated in the spectacle, ultimately sharing in the enactment. The self-containment and privilege that set the viewer apart from the characters and the events on stage are stripped away by a dramatization that refuses to pander to the viewer's will to guard his privilege as a spectator whose isolation shelters him from the plot that unfolds onstage. Whatever private thoughts and feelings the drama engenders in the spectator become, in this way, public and shared.

In an odd turn of events, however, the play suffered various abuses at the hands of censors, as it raised a storm of protest in the puritan and bourgeois circles of London. Its derivation from an imperial Orientalist tradition, "drawing on contemporary obsessions with the East, and notions of oriental cruelty" (Hoare 72), could not rescue it from censorship by the Lord Chamberlain's office. When it was prohibited by the censor, the play was already in full rehearsal by Sarah Bernhardt at the Palace Theatre (Ross 15). The biblical references were sufficient qualification for banning its performance, although the Dance of the Seven Veils, as "a key marker for the transgressive interweaving of sexuality and the sacred" (Deagon, "Dance of the Seven Veils" 1), instrumented the play's particularly hostile handling, and lasting ridicule by some. It is no accident that Salomé should be the archetype to invoke an ideological obsession among the decadents. As the iconic "new woman," she formed the counterpart to the decadent male aesthete, both challenging the institution of marriage and blurring the borders between the sexes (Showalter 169).[1] In Wilde's treatment, however, the princess retained her exoticism, her excess, her bejewelled seduction, and yet she transcended the confines of du Camp's uncertain, narrow, and colonizing attraction. She became a character of compelling passion who imbued the entire theatrical space (stage and orchestra) with her "excess and transgression." In a sense, Wilde's Salomé colonizes the metropolitan space itself, imposing in the imperial realm her lexicon of desire and her economy of passion.

114

*Dancing
Decadence:
Semiotics
of Dance
and the
Phantasm of
Salmomé*

Dance, Sex, and Salomé Go to Court

On 3 September 1895, four "exotic" dancers who were performing at the Coney Island sideshows (one of them was, apparently, Farehda Mahzar, who is the most likely contestant for the title of the legendary "Little Egypt") were arrested following a police raid.[2] The Oriental dancers performing at the Turkish theatre were deemed immoral and offensive and the arrests were intended, it seems, to alert the people to the moral pitfalls in the entertainment. Police intervention also aimed at stopping the assault on public propriety and encouraging the moral edification of the entertainment offered at the amusement park. Paul Eugene Monty informs us that while in court, upon the advice of their lawyer, they danced for the judge and jury so that the law could decide upon the morality of the dance (106)!

This ludicrous procedure feigns ignorance about the nature and politics of performance, expecting the performance in court to replicate the "real" performance when the context and the dynamics are vastly different. But what is important about the courtroom story is that the litigation against dance and dancers strongly parallels legislation on sexuality and, more specifically, the spectacle of homosexual sex. As queer sexuality contradicts the norm, Middle Eastern dance contradicts proper posture and upsets respectability. Across the Atlantic, and in the same year that Oriental dance was performed in court at Coney Island, Oscar Wilde's sexual encounters in male brothels were narrated and made into spectacle during the trials that ended with his two-year sentence at hard labour. Wilde served his sentence at Reading, condemned under the same Labouchere Amendment Act that also determined the sexual behaviour of the Cypriots and, by extension, their performance of sexuality and gender. It seems to me that Wilde's sentence as political development, Salomé as aesthetic embodiment, and on-going colonial politics converge tragically in the *fin de siècle*. In a sense, the ending of the play foreshadows Wilde's own downfall. When Salomé bends to kiss the mouth of the beheaded saint, Herod observes her necrophilic gesture and judges her to be perverted and monstrous. Instantly, he orders his soldiers to crush Salomé to death. Wilde's is the only version of the story "to terminate in the little princess being put to death for her alleged depravity by someone who is arguably more corrupt than she herself" (Ellis 55). Through her death she becomes herself a martyr victimized for her passion, and she expires, ironically, over a beheaded ascetic.

Oscar Wilde's conviction, however, did not signal the end of litigations over Wilde, Salomé, and the "veiled dance." Towards the end of the First World War, another trial took place—a trial once more directly related to performances of gender, sex, and empire. In London, in the winter of 1917, Maud Allan, a Canadian dancer from Toronto, accepted the lead role in Wilde's play. J.T. Grein, a drama critic for the reputable *Sunday Times* and one of Allan's foremost admirers, was instrumental in offering her the part. According to Felix Cherniavsky, Grein was also the driving force behind a theatre society interested in staging mostly modern and controversial plays before private audiences. The privacy of the performances exempted the Independent Theatre Society from the Lord Chamberlain's censorship (Cherniavsky 240). *Salomé* had never seen a public performance in England before this time and it appeared that this particular society was ideal for staging the play by "the most publicly disgraced Decadent" (Cherniavsky 240) and featuring a dancer who had visited Wilde in Paris shortly before his death (242).

Following the advertisement for the performance in April 1918, an independent MP, Noel Pemberton Billing, editor of a weekly political broadsheet, *The Vigilante*, published a deliberately provocative but cryptic paragraph entitled "The Cult of the Clitoris" (Hawthorne 159, Cherniavsky 242, Hoare 90-92). The headline was indeed "salacious," as Philip Hoare points out, yet "the salacity was lost on most of its readers, few of whom knew the meaning of the term [clitoris]" (91). The readers may have been ignorant of what "clitoris" meant, yet they were clearly informed about a certain list numbering 47,000 "depraved" individuals. These people were, supposedly, guilty of being disloyal, unpatriotic citizens, enemies of their own country. Pemberton's publication stirred the nationalistic feelings of its readership by directly suggesting that those individuals who intended to house Maud Allan's "private performances [of] Oscar Wilde's *Salomé*" were among the dishonourable enemies of the state: "If Scotland Yard were to seize the list of these members I have no doubt they would secure the names of several of the first 47,000" (qtd. in Hoare 91). As Melanie Hawthorne puts it, "the article may as well have accused Allen [*sic*] of 'posing as a somdomite [*sic*]' as the Marquess of Queensberry had said of Wilde. Allen filed suit for libel, along with J.T. Grein ... and a curious reprise of the 1895 trials took place" (159). In the litigation that ensued, what was dragged through court, by a nearly hysterical system, was deviant sexuality. Not only was it an abomination, it was decidedly unpatriotic. This enemy sexuality met its avatar in the

116

Dancing
Decadence:
Semiotics
of Dance
and the
Phantasm of
Salmomé

body of a depraved dance performance. Once again, Wilde, dance, and deviant sexuality were conflated into a symbol which, this time, became particularly useful in rallying against various kinds of purported political corruptions and bolstering national sentiment about the war. "In a word," Hawthorne argues, "the trial once again made Wilde's body (of work) the site of a debate between expression of sexuality and the national interest" (160). Allan and Grein lost the case. Such was the nationalist sentiment, and so delicate were the public's moral pretensions, that there was no room for accepting a barefoot dancer's rendition of a heretic's dance as it was written by Oscar Wilde, whose sexual proclivities qualified him as a heretic also.

Interestingly, when it came to interpretations of *Salomé*, Maud Allan was not a novice. She had performed the part in the past, yet the history of these performances reveals the cautious ideological balancing required of this particular performance, and also the inevitable complications that invariably resulted from it. In 1908, Allan's production of *The Vision of Salomé* enjoyed enormous success at the Palace Theatre in London. Amy Koritz posits that, performing the fantasy of the Eastern woman, *Salomé* was an "ideologically unstable event requiring the careful manipulation of available vocabularies in order to keep the overlapping and mutually reinforcing categories of Western and native clearly distinct" ("Dancing the Orient" 133). Allan's dancing in this particular version relied for its success on "an interaction of racial and gender stereotyping that reinforced English assumptions about the 'Oriental.' This Orientalism (in Said's sense of the term) in turn depended upon a rhetoric that characterized as female those attributes that denoted the inferiority of England's colonized peoples" (Koritz, "Dancing the Orient" 133).[3]

When Salomé's dance, therefore, departed from the pages of the Scriptures to assume centre position on the metropolitan stage, it had to be transformed into something acceptable. Although for the performer it may have had lofty incentives, the outcome was often to reinforce existing stereotypes of abject, racially inferior others. For example, in Flaubert's short story "Herodias," the dance scene occupies a proportionately large space and is depicted with particular detail. However, as Andrea Deagon argues in her article "The Image of the Easter Dancer: Flaubert's Salomé," in translating the spectacle for his short story, "his Salomé does not have the flawed individuality of the Eastern dancers he admired but the iconic beauty appropriate for the Western stage" (14). Kuchuk's incisor going bad and Hassan el-Balbeissi's ugliness, for example, qualify for this "flawed individuality" that Flaubert eschews in his literary creation. He declares Salomé's dance to be "Oriental": "She danced like the priestesses of the Indies, like the Nubian girls of the cataracts, like the bacchantes of Lydia," yet she also "pirouetted madly round the Tetrarch's table" ("Herodias" 121). Following a close reading of the dance scene, Deagon concludes that what Salomé performed was a Western version of Eastern dance—a version that Oriental dancers still use today: "The balletic Orientalisms of Flaubert's Salomé fit Oriental dancers like a glove and we are often unable even to recognize them" (Deagon, "Image of the Easter Dancer" 15).

Decadence as a movement responded to imperial pursuits during what Ali Behdad calls "the age of colonial dissolution"—the time, in other words, when disciples of Orientalism participated in an exoticist exploration of a topography that had already been mapped and familiarized as a site of Western hegemony. As a result, "these Orientalists could not help but experience a sense of displacement in time and space, an experience that produced either a sense of disorientation and loss or an obsessive urge to discover an 'authentic' Other" (Behdad 13). With Salomé as exotic ecphrasis, there was no fear of temporal or topographic displacement. She did not reside in Wadi Halfa, like Kuchuk Hanem, and she did not make appearances at Mousky coffee houses like the khawals or at the taverns of Galata like the koçek. Yet she was strangely "authentic" in her polyvalence, with all her incarnations offering themselves genuinely to a sexual or aesthetic purpose of their creation. The decadent Salomé, then, is a Middle Eastern dancer tailored to the heterogeneous needs of a Europe that has exhausted itself yearning for an Orient.

As with Flaubert, in Wilde's play, Salomé is an alien, a dancing and scandalous body, just as the Middle East is. However, Wilde's treatment presents a novel and daring configuration. He stages her excess through a number of decadent references, from allusions to green flowers (supposedly worn by Parisian homosexuals), "to the metaphorical moon hanging over the proceedings, a decadent perversion of the more normal poetic use of the sun" (Hoare 72). As Garelick conceives it, Wilde's objective relates aptly to the dynamics of Middle Eastern dance:

> Wilde consistently undermines exclusive possession of or dominion over riches, a love object, personality, language, or even one's own gaze. In Salomé, all are subsumed by the chorus and the crowd. The rarified is no longer set off from the common. Wilde flings open the door to a highly ornate closet, and the surprise is that we are all inside it. (129)

118

*Dancing
Decadence:
Semiotics
of Dance
and the
Phantasm of
Salmomé*

In the same way that the Middle Eastern dancer involves the viewer, the play does not allow for any false security of spectatorship. Salomé provokes the need to be possessed, transitively and intransitively, a body whose movement and sound are more a theatrical enactment of our phobias, desires, and fascinations (even though the dancing body is non-verbal, it resonates in an aesthetically sonic dimension so we need to hear it as well as see it). Her performance is so much a reflection of the audience's apocryphal passions that no distance, physical or emotional, can offer adequate protection from the spectacle. In choreographed kinesthesia the phantasm of what is danced incarnates in the observer's eyes, exacting a response in the dialogue it initiates.

Wilde, who liked to think of his life as Art, moved in a constant yet perilous and foreboding dance as he performed the dandy, the heterosexual husband and father, the queer lover, and the decadent, hedonistic homosexual. But his performance of Britishness or Irishness was a different issue and one that set Wilde apart from established nationalist politics. In a brilliant discussion of nationalism and sexuality, Eve Sedgwick asserts that Wilde embodied his sexual identity radically. The exotic is erotic, but then so is "the domestic Same," Sedgwick argues (*Tendencies* 150). Wilde's homosexual imagining of same-sex desire did not rely exclusively on a definition of Englishness against the overseas Empire:

> Wilde, as an ambitious Irishman, and the son, intimate, and protégé of a celebrated Irish nationalist poet, can only have had as a fundamental element of his own sense of self an exquisitely exacerbated sensitivity to how by turns porous, brittle, elastic, chafing, embracing, exclusive, murderous, in every way contestable and contested were the membranes of "domestic" national definition signified by the ductile and elusive terms England, Britain, Ireland. (151)

Wilde and Salomé embodied the very attribute that national definition relies upon—difference. And it was, paradoxically, in this difference that male-male desire, "based on sameness" (151), came alive. He foregrounded his longing in his body "so insistently as an index to such erotic and political meanings" (151). His *Salomé*, then, as I have tried to illustrate (with a lot of help from Rhonda Garelick), is not so much about the West desiring the exotic Orient but about desiring the exotic Occident. The oxymoron conceals but also reveals itself in the image of the veiled dancer. The dance is an aesthetic palliative, codifying desire in terms that may obscure and detract from the play's scope. Yet, as an existing art form with a particular vocabulary of moves (shimmies, hip drops, undulations, and so on) and a geographical point of reference (the Middle East), the dance reveals this brand of desire. Salomé moves in the veils Wilde invested himself and dances to her death, sustaining her challenging configurations. Through her kinesthetic excess, she appears to signal that Middle Eastern dance cannot pledge the purity of a distinct gendered space.

This unique space of dance has been described by Judith Lynne Hanna in *Dance, Sex, and Gender,* where she attempts a definition of dance that concludes with the interesting suggestion that "dance exists in three dimensions of space, one of time, and another in the realm of imagination" (46). I believe that this realm is where the body dances and where the observer meets the dancer. The imagination is the region of intercourse between viewer and dancer, yet this intercourse also enjoys a purely physical fulfillment, hence the phobia that characterizes approaches to Middle Eastern dance. These comments anticipate my following chapter on the Greek politics of dance and the choreophobic attempts to curtail its influence and to restructure dance discourse in the eager hope that Greece could leave its ambivalent—and therefore anxious—condition and move as close to the metropolitan centre as this construction could take it. Salomé is a formidable figure for the orthodox Greek imaginary, as she suggests pagan dissipation, unspeakable unions, passions, and an unbridled, and therefore, irresistible, Orientalist excess.

5 / "I have seen this dance on old Greek vases"
Hellenism and the Worlding of Greek Dance

Lord Valencia describes the dances of Cairo as being too lascivious even for description. Mrs. Macarolle, a pretty Greek, was present, with a number of ladies, at an entertainment where his lordship was; they looked on without the least discomposure, and thought so little from habit of its impropriety, that, when asked, they danced themselves with the same motions and gestures.

Lady Augusta Hamilton, *Marriage, Rites, Customs and Ceremonies of All Nations of the Universe*

The value of utilizing folk dance for the representation of an entire nation emanates from the common public view that these dances emerge from some primordial source of the nation's purest and most authentic values and that folk dances, music and costumes are timeless and date from some prehistoric period.

Anthony Shay, *Choreographic Politics: State Folk Dance Ensembles, Representation, and Power*

In the Orthodox Church of a diasporic Greek community (vaguely) located in the upper Midwest, Angela Shand experienced an actual "Tsifte-teli Sermon." This sermon took place on a Sunday following a Greek celebration, which the local priest supported by encouraging his flock to attend. Following the event, the community priest sombrely announced that "he felt betrayed," as he had publicly supported this event without having been told about the belly dancing that opened the show.

 Notes to chapter 5 are on page 211.

"I have seen
this dance on
old Greek
vases":
Hellenism
and the
Worlding of
Greek Dance

The priest went on to say that "this type of dancing led to sin: Salomé herself had danced in this manner and enticed King Herod to behead John the Baptist. Furthermore, he added, tsifte-teli is not even a Greek folk dance, but of Turkish origin, and therefore should not be danced or enjoyed by Greeks" (Shand 128).

My analysis in the previous chapters has examined colonial attitudes to the dancing body, especially the distinct anxieties engendered by male and female performers in the Middle East. My efforts concentrated on ascertaining the extent to which these anxieties forged the images that Western imperialism desired to be abhorred, charmed, and captivated by. Ultimately, the phobias of the Eastern dancing body lie in the potential of any body to perform the derided movements—a possibility that provokes both perverse pleasure and dismay. In this chapter, I will extend the discussion to the dances "on old Greek vases" and the contemporary politics of "Eastern" dance in an attempt to map some of the processes through which the exchange dynamic between East and West enacts itself within the disputed Greek cultural borders. These processes have been closely influenced by Greek political developments on the national and international level. However, the "Greece" I am concerned with is not only the modern geographical state but also the nationalist construct that dominates the consciousness of Hellenic-identified communities and individuals, both at home and in the diaspora. In line with my overall scope, I will focus specifically on the tsifteteli and the anxieties elicited by its "Oriental" associations. These hark back to the Ottoman occupation of Greece that lasted nearly four centuries—a chapter in the nation's history that is recounted as the most bitter and hurtful—yet they also relate to the fervent desire for a modern Greek identity that is completely unconnected with the Orient and firmly identifies, instead, with European civilization.

My discussion consists mainly of two parts. I will examine the politics inherent in Dora Stratou's national folkloric dance company. This examination will, I hope, yield some understanding of the manner in which her ambitious project achieved its overwhelming effects, namely the rewriting of dance traditions in modern Greece, which have been instituted as the "living museum" of Greek culture. Second, I will look at the effects of the influx of refugees from Asia Minor on Greek cultural developments. They brought with them a cultural heritage whose elements were decidedly "Oriental," with the tsifteteli as an integral part of these people's dance expression. The tragic historical events that forced these populations to flee their homes in Western Turkey in 1922 played a significant part in twentieth-century cultural politics, and had a profound impact on Greek musical production. I want to examine the tsifteteli in relation to the zeibekiko, another solo improvisational dance made popular in Greece by the fleeing refugees. In parts of Greece, especially the islands, in Cyprus and in Turkey, there exist various folkloric renditions of the zeibekiko. In Cyprus, the most popular version is the "azizies," although there exist others, which are sometimes strictly regional too. When I refer to the zeibekiko in this project, however, I mean the urban, rebetiko rendition that is performed mostly solo, and in my examination of it I hope to delineate ways in which the Greek dance scene, much like the Egyptian (and the Turkish), has been and continues to be a stage where Orientalism and Occidentalism compete in a contest where the rules can neither be obeyed nor ignored. Nevertheless, the imperative antagonism within this binary is what determines the performances of ethnic identity, masculinity, femininity, and sexuality in the Greek context. The movements of the tsifteteli unsettle these performances, instigating a tension that becomes a form of counter-hegemonic discourse-in-motion.

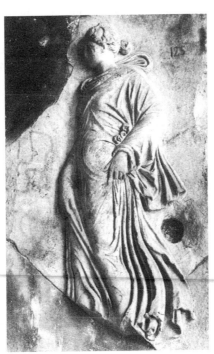

Relief of a Dancing Girl. 1915. From the collection of the National Archaeological Museum of Athens. (Reprinted with permission from *Dance 1900: Greek Turn-of-the-Century Postcards Portraying Dance* by Alkis Raftis.)

"I have seen
this dance on
old Greek
vases":
Hellenism
and the
Worlding of
Greek Dance

Hellenism and Cultural Etiquette

As we saw in chapter 1, political events and decision making in Cyprus of the 1950s were closely connected to crucial political developments in Greece. The Nazi occupation of Greece was a time of great hardship for the people and great population loss. Yet the horrors unfortunately repeated themselves in the aftermath of the war. Those who did not perish from famine, in the fighting against the German forces, or from Nazi retaliation against the resistance lived through the horrors of a civil war that followed the Nazi occupation. This four-year civil war between the communist-led Greek resistance and the monarchy and military elite was fought to determine not only Greek rule but essentially Greece's political affiliations in the immediate future. Marked by massacres and mass executions, the horrifying civil war burned a painful and lasting scar in the bodies, memory, and culture of the survivors. As one would anticipate, considering the catalytic British and American role in world affairs, the outcome of the Greek conflict owed a great deal to the allies, whose main concerns included the prevention of communist control or influence in Greece. Their victory became consolidated not only politically, by making Greece a British protectorate, but also ideologically. The wave of nationalism that swept Greece furthered the rise of imperialism in the country.[1] Nationalism quite obviously linked itself to Western ideals yet it also aspired for the political security that Western allegiances seemed to promise.

In travel narratives, Greece often constituted "a little corner of the Orient" but also "a little corner of Europe" although, overwhelmingly, Greeks were termed "uncivilized" and "tribal" in their manners and customs, and often discursively referred to by the West in purely Orientalist terms (Peckham 171). George William Curtis's description of Kuchuk Hanem in terms of Terpsichore (see chapter 2), the ancient Greek dance muse, relies on ambivalence for effect. In the minds of Curtis's learned readers, Terpsichore was likely to evoke an ethereal and lofty image of classical art but also an identification of Greece with the exotic Orient. This identification is also what prompted Flaubert to observe Kuchuk's dance on ancient Greek vases. In an interesting foray into Greek dance during the Ottoman years, Alkis Raftis draws attention to and identifies some misunderstandings that have occurred in the interpretation of a number of Greek dance traditions. Raftis explains that foreign travellers to Greece insist on the inevitable comparisons of their contemporary experience of the culture with the ancient Greeks. Every dance with knives

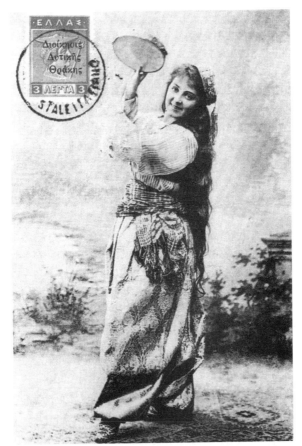

"Salonica–Oriental dancer." 1910. The caption situates the photograph in Chania (on Crete) but this might not be necessarily the case. It has also circulated with a caption from Salonica. This type of photograph featuring professional dancers was very popular at the time. The dancer's sash and gold-threaded fez with golden tassel are typical of urban costumes from centres such as Ioannina, Veroia, and Athens. (Comments by Alkis Raftis. My translation. Reprinted with permission from *Dance 1900: Greek Turn-of-the-Century Postcards Portraying Dance* by Alkis Raftis.)

or sharp moves is certainly the ancient "Pyrrihios," every dance where the young women hold handkerchiefs is the dance of Ariadne, and so on. Most interesting, perhaps, is Raftis's comment that when the cultural event could not be readily linked to the ancient past, the foreign tourist would find the dances boring and the music despairingly cacophonic (*The World of Hellenic Dance* 36).[2] In other words, Orientalist discourse would take the place of classical glories and Greece would become, in those disengaged passages, the Oriental, uncivilized land.

"I have seen
this dance on
old Greek
vases":
Hellenism
and the
Worlding of
Greek Dance

Greece's significance for the West, however, was not merely cultural but also sexual. When Lord Byron, a British elite and an erudite classicist, travelled and resided there, it was not merely as a fervent supporter of Romantic Hellenism. Greece offered him what Italy was unable to: an Oriental setting and "flavour" complete with ruthless, savage, and noble rulers with an insolent sexual appetite, such as Ali Pasha of Ioannina, as well as visible remnants of Europe's classical past.[3] Prominent in Byron's Orientalist experience was the anticipation of homosexual encounters. Ali Pasha himself was, apparently, a lover of young boys and the court that accommodated, literally and metaphorically, his sexual predilections formed an alluring centre for Byron. Greece seemed to promise the British poet shelter from Georgian homophobia. At the same time, it permitted indulgence in homoerotic pleasures that were characteristically Oriental in European discourse, hence Byron's contribution to and focus on neo-Hellenism and not merely on the ghosts of classical antiquity.[4]

Aware of such constructions and with the legacy of the Ottoman occupation prominent in the culture and their architectural landscape, those Greeks who could settle for a share in an "Oriental" identity remedied their own discomfort by accepting a location on the cusp of East and West. Officially, however, the modern state has been prepared to denounce any ostensibly "Eastern" heritage in an anxious attempt to secure Western allegiances. Often this denunciation was an act that amounted to nothing less than a cultural self-mutilation, since a great deal of Greek culture qualifies as "Eastern." The aphoristic treatment of music produced by the Asia Minor refugees (music known as "rebetika") provides a paradigm of the cultural mutilation, a paradigm I will return to in the final section of this chapter.[5] Even the Greek Orthodox Church, which has played a catalytic and also oppressive role in the creation of cultural, political and individual character, is an Eastern Church. In fact, Byzantium was instrumental in the formation of the Greek and Turkish musical traditions. Therefore, the ideology by which Greece came to denounce any influences that denoted a geographical East wreaked havoc in Greek cultural affairs and it informs a crisis that seems to rage even now in varying degrees wherever Greek populations live.

Michael Herzfeld identifies the Greek elite as having a significant share in this cultural overhaul of modern Greece:

> The Greeks were effectively taught that whatever was most familiar in their everyday lives was probably of Turkish origin and therefore by definition "foreign." The local, largely occidentalized élite eagerly enforced this

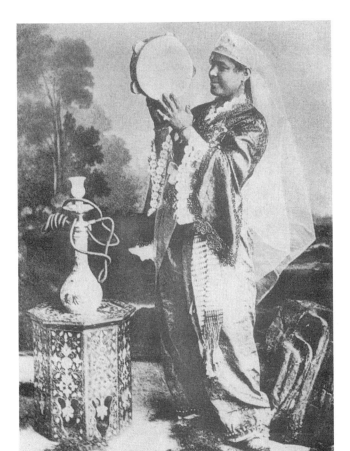

"Smyrna; Paysanne en costume de danse." 1905. Professional dancers of the time were often Greek and more rarely Armenian or Jewish. This photo does not depict "a village girl in a dancer's outfit" as the caption reads. Her costume is of the Eastern urban style established by the Ottoman court of Constantinople. The card was mailed to Glasgow from the British post office at Smyrna. (Comments by Alkis Raftis. My translation. Reprinted with permission from *Dance 1900: Greek Turn-of-the-Century Postcards Portraying Dance* by Alkis Raftis.)

process of cultural cleansing, since its own relatively secure access to philological classicism—enshrined in its use of the puristic *katharevousa* (i.e., "cleansed") language—gave it practical advantages to which it subsequently clung in the realistic assessment that this cultural etiquette also secured its monopoly of power and wealth. ("Hellenism and Occidentalism" 218-19)

Knowledge of classical philology and an investment in privilege made the elite class the most appropriate to cultivate the passion for the glo-

"I have seen
this dance on
old Greek
vases":
Hellenism
and the
Worlding of
Greek Dance

rious past. "Progonoplexia" (Προγονοπληξία), or "excessive worship of the ancestors" (Shay, *Choreographic Politics* 254) was the most intriguing component of the elite's fabrication of modern Greece. Of course, the choice of ancestors to worship is quite telling of the motivations and also the aspirations underlying this movement. This choice involved a persistent and systematic denial of Ottoman associations and even a wilful ignorance of the cultural opulence of Byzantine heritage. Instead, what came to propel Modern Greek aspirations was an ideological fetishization of the legacy of classical Greece. As I indicate in my introduction, this fetishization had formed the staple diet of Western Europe's intellectual and elite populations, hence its necessary appeal for the modern Greeks.

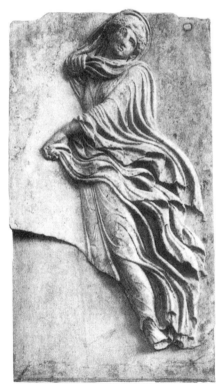

"Athenes–Danseuse." 1900. One of the first cards depicting themes from Ancient Greece intended for the foreign tourists to Athens. The representation is of a female dancer on a plaque discovered in 1862 at the Theatre of Dionysus. This is a sample of 2nd century BC Attic art and possibly a copy of a 4th century piece. The dancer's right hand is holding the gown that covers her body. (Comments by Alkis Raftis. My translation. Reprinted with permission from *Dance 1900: Greek Turn-of-the-Century Postcards Portraying Dance*.)

129

Dora Stratou
and the
Construction
of Greek
Folklore

Dora Stratou and the Construction of Greek Folklore

Dora Stratou carried through this classical legacy in the field of dance. She was the founder of the first national Greek dance ensemble, a project that materialized because of her hard work and persistence but also because of ideological affiliations, government connections, and wealthy artistic and intellectual supporters. Almost single-handedly, she led a crusade to retrieve, rescue, and bring to the forefront what was the vanquished cultural grandeur of classical Greece, according to a conviction she shared with the ruling authorities. Her project was propelled by a phobia that modern Greece would be "Orientalized" under Western eyes, a prospect so horrifying that it directed her efforts with a hysterical hand. In her perception, this grandeur and high artistic achievement were not lost but simply lay dormant through the "dark centuries" of Ottoman occupation. Undertaking a long and laborious project, she researched and catalogued Greek traditional costumes and folk dances from the entire Greek countryside, omitting songs in languages other than Greek, and presented the sum of her efforts in spectacular shows intended to dazzle Greeks with this rediscovery of their identity. In an enterprise whose success was predictable considering the dominant rhetoric, Stratou served Greek audiences an exoticized and therefore commercialized spectacle of what they were told was their heritage. Indeed, the commodification and exploitation of dance for ideological purposes found in Dora Stratou a most triumphant exponent. Her conviction that contemporary Greek dances could be directly traced to ancient customs and dance events engendered an irresistible appeal in the reactionary circles of Greece in the latter half of the 1960s.

In pursuing such ideological constructs, Stratou added her name to a long line of classical enthusiasts and proponents of the "grandeur" that was Greece, but she was also perpetuating a discourse that would prove useful to the fascist regime of 1967-1974. When her argument materialized in a book entitled *The Greek Dances: Our Living Link with Antiquity*, published in 1966, the Greek government, eager to perpetuate the same ideals and cultivate a sense of nationalism and identity that were firmly rooted in a glorified and idealistic vision of Greece, reprinted and distributed free copies of her project to schools (Pizanias 25).[6] At the time, the quality of Stratou's argument or of her scholarship went unchallenged and their value was undisputed. Caterina Pizanias finds Stratou's efforts in the book to be "at best rather impressionistic and at worst naïve and misleading, for [Stratou] assumes that some photographs of ancient reliefs

"I have seen
this dance on
old Greek
vases":
Hellenism
and the
Worlding of
Greek Dance

and vases, along with quotes from Homer, Plutarch, and Xenophon, convincingly support her alleged 'living' connection" (27). Moreover, it seems that the passion itself that propelled Stratou in her work belongs to the category of "emotional capital" that, as Marta Savigliano argues, rises out of an "imperialist circulation of feelings" (2). In other words, Stratou's fervent wish to excavate the site of Greek culture and sift through layers and layers of cultural debris only to discover some pristine form right there on the surface is yet another articulation of nationalist rhetoric. In fact, her efforts were connected to, and in a sense empowered by, her right-wing affiliations and her government connections, something that is now openly talked about in Greece (contrary to the silence of the 1960s and '70s on such issues).

Stratou's endeavours acquire an interesting dimension when examined under the rubric of "auto-exoticization," a term that derives from Mary Louise Pratt's concept of "autoethnographic expression." Such expression, Pratt explains, is "an instance in which colonized subjects undertake to represent themselves in ways that *engage with* the colonizer's own terms" (7). Stratou's search for origins and authenticity, and the confident and triumphant tracing of origins to a historical, glorious past, is a component of the colonizing project that seeks to establish an identity for the uncivilized, primitive, and inept present. In the case of Dora Stratou, however, the exoticization happens from within the culture and is embedded in the operation that strives to reimport what is perceived as the inherent (that is, classical civilization) to the domestic (that is, contemporary) Greek culture. Christian Zervos wrote the introduction to *The Greek Dances: Our Living Link with Antiquity*, where he asserts emphatically that,

> the spectacle Dora Stratou has offered us these past many years embraces only those dances whose authenticity is absolutely guaranteed. For Dora Stratou is interested only in the dances for which she finds crystal-clear evidence. These dances as they are still danced today are precious, for they have preserved their original movements in their entirety. And the tremendous value of Dora Stratou is that she has succeeded in showing us this choreography absolutely unaltered, with all its archaic elements intact. She is convinced that what many of the so-called "popular" dances are incapable of carrying off, the authentic dances can assume the responsibility of recalling to us. (8)

While strongly affirming the valence of Stratou's project, which he takes as undisputable, Zervos's declaration also insinuates an incompleteness

131

*Dora Stratou
and the
Construction
of Greek
Folklore*

and lack of homogeny (ομογένεια) in the group's national identity. In a gesture that supports and enhances the goals of Stratou's project, he refers with a certain disdain to the "so-called 'popular dances'" that obviously lack genuine tradition and proper identity. (There is little doubt that the tsifteteli would take its place in this suspicious category of misleading "popular" dances.) In this way, Zervos joins Stratou in setting up a dichotomy of Greek cultural contemporaneity, distinguishing between the proper and the inauthentic, in an attitude that somehow delivers a subtle admonition to the public that does not value what Stratou's project has salvaged. Moreover, Stratou expects us to see our contemporary identity reflected in our classical past and, further, our obligation is to recognize and acknowledge the roots of this identity. Of course, Stratou poses as the luminary who will show us the way. She condescends to acknowledge that Greeks "naturally enough, were not aware of the significance of their dances and their songs" (35). Following this concession to popular ignorance, which is reminiscent of the infantilization that became a standard trope in the representation of colonized peoples, she then assigns a role of resistance to the festivals organized during the years of Ottoman occupation. These celebrations were "the only way [Greeks] could come together without giving the conqueror grounds for suspicion" (35). Bringing up the duress of slavery under the Ottoman conqueror further fortifies her blackmail to secure more labour to operate her ideological machinery.

Stratou explains how, following the Greek war of independence—which lasted from 1821 to 1828—the Greeks emerged out of four centuries of Turkish enslavement. Turkey is "an eastern power," she emphasizes, and the Greeks, eager to relieve themselves of this burden, "longed to approach the West with which so many ties from the past linked them" (35). It was contrapuntal readings of such imperialist teachings that made me realize the imperative for a decolonization project. This passage in her text is one of those moments that made discernible to me how the Greeks and Greek Cypriots came to observe the dances of the East through a Western gaze, despite the fact that these dances still occupy an ambiguous position in the East/West binary. They hover in a constantly shifting state within the collective cultural imagination.

This complex process of auto-exoticization also makes an imperative contribution to the instituting and subsequent adherence to an "exclusive axis of allowed versus forbidden national articulations" (Gourgouris 13). This axis may not always take the form of legislative action,

"I have seen
this dance on
old Greek
vases":
Hellenism
and the
Worlding of
Greek Dance

yet its existence hovers and polices the various individual behaviours, especially the corporeal. An implementation of this policing takes place through a certain blackmail mechanism that installs itself in the Greek psyche. It activates itself, often surreptitiously, in the form of an austere ethical self-interrogation that takes over whenever a subject decides to challenge or disobey Stratou's construct that we are direct descendants of the ancient Greeks and that our lineage is embodied in the performance of our dances.[7] In a passage that extols Greek presence (and, according to this logic, prerogative as well) in various regions around the Mediterranean Sea, she sketches roughly and simplistically the parameters of Greekdom. She asserts that, even though the geography of Greek control may have shifted, Greek values have remained immutable:

> There have been Greeks both in the area known as present day Greece and in Asia Minor, definitely ever since the eighth century BC: the time when Hellenism spread beyond the borders and began founding colonies along all the coasts of Asia Minor, crossing the straits of the Hellespont to found Byzantium in 660 BC.... Primitive peoples, pugnacious and barbarous—Turks, Slavs, Bulgarians, Arabs and others—swept down into our land from the late sixth century AD on, striking at the Empire both from the East and the North. And some of them, e.g., the Bulgarians, remained here ever since. This is yet another proof of their having been influenced by our dances and our ancient musical meter and the ancient Greek scales; and moreover, by many of our customs, costumes, embroidery motifs, which have passed over to them in corrupted form and which we can still see to this very day. And thus, they still have deep roots in the prototypes of our own ancestors: a crystal clear proof of the survival of our own element. (33-34)

Such declarations distill a certain epistemology of "Hellenism" that for decades now has been made the staple diet of school children in the Greek part of Cyprus where I grew up and in several (if not all) parts of Greece. The most immediately recognizable characteristics of this epistemology are its confidence and its masking of romanticism by substantiating the arguments with supposedly undisputed historical facts. The blackmail I referred to earlier is suggested by the very threads that weave this ideological construct. By fabricating the overtly racist image of barbaric and uncivilized Others overriding Greek nobility, this rhetoric manipulates the modern Greek subject into subscribing to this belief; otherwise s/he will be abandoned as a race traitor who identifies with the non-Hellenic hordes.

Writing about Stratou's venture, Smaro Kamboureli critiques the staging of folklore for diasporic communities and draws attention to the ultimate exclusion of the very subjects whom the project claims to represent. Her comments are relevant to many of the points I have tried to make:

> Folklore, then, is employed both to obscure and to reveal. Endorsed and promoted as the most transparent form of cultural authenticity, it can also lead to cultural insiderism, an absolute belief in essential differences. It encourages and feeds the sort of nostalgia that results in cultural mutation, locking ethnic subjects between "here" and "there" while feigning to resolve their fragmentation. Thus even as it affords them the opportunity to celebrate and share their heritage, it detemporalizes them, creating the semblance of historical continuity, in effect a form of hegemonic modernity. (107)

Dora Stratou's initiative, then, was no initiative at all. It was more her immense and unparalleled subscription to "hegemonic modernity," a selective rescuing from the ravages of time of those elements of folk culture which can be manipulated to elicit a certain nostalgia, that ultimately divides and detemporalizes modern subjects. What has been discarded, such as dances to songs with lyrics in Turkish, Albanian, Bulgarian, and Vlach languages (Shay, *Choreographic Politics* 270), may not have vanished completely but continued some course in an "anachronistic space." Stratou's work was a transformative project that served a more immediate ideological expedient with direct political implications. Invited to pose as a glorious albeit vague and ill-defined ideal, the ancient past was revived as the only appropriate donor of identity.

One of the most "charming" and also revelatory moments in Dora Stratou's *The Greek Dances* is her reference to a (male) dancer's evidently improvisational moment. Apparently, she feels that such moments require some explication since the dancer seems to be getting out of control and is about to threaten the viewer with the discomfort of transgressive movement. My need to focus on this moment stems from the connection I discern between these moves and the general perception of the tsifteteli and, more specifically, the kinesthetics that reify this dance. Stratou offers a facile resolution of that potentially uncomfortable moment when the dancer, in a solo aside, seems to succumb to the influence of damaging demons:

> One of the most characteristic points of Greek dancing, as far as its "Greekness" goes, is the following: however intense a dance may be, even if it is

134

"I have seen
this dance on
old Greek
vases":
Hellenism
and the
Worlding of
Greek Dance

steadily accelerating its rhythm, it *never* goes beyond the proper limits.... You may see a dancer growing more and more excited, more and more dionysiac—And you think to yourself: "Where can this possibly wind up?"—Well, the dancer simply stops and sits down calmly. At the very most, he may be highly pleased with his own accomplishments as a dancer. The "golden mean" prevails, the "golden mean" of the ancients. Balance in all things—Harmony. (34)

Whom is Dora Stratou addressing in this telling passage and what and whose fears is she trying to assuage? I discern in Stratou's exposition a contribution to the process of *embourgeoisement* of dance, the same Foucauldian term that Edward Said uses to mark the developments in the nineteenth-century discourse on sex (*Orientalism* 180). She is eager to reassure her audience that any behaviour that could be termed "excessive," and thereby threatening to the established order, is absent from Greek performance. Stratou's attempt is to tame the dance and divest it of any potential for personal, as opposed to national, expression, because in her philosophy dance has to be practised with control. Without circumspection it will go beyond all degrees of propriety, shunning modesty and restraint.[8] Underlying her comments I also hear the bourgeois anxiety regarding the dancer's transgressive potential. Clearly, Stratou needs to desexualize the dance, since the moment of solo improvisation is the moment of initiative and private artistic expression calling for attention to the individual dancer's body. So, to return to the question of who is being addressed in this passage: I think it is a pre-emptive gesture directed at both the dancer and the viewer, ultimately aimed at pacifying and directing both—the dancer must not perform excessive movement and interpret the dance "untameably" (as Marta Savigliano would put it) and the viewer must not be apprehensive in the anticipation of embarrassing corporeal excess because the dancer will simply, in the end, sit down balanced, calm, and harmonious.

In Anthony Shay's terms, Stratou's silencing of the dancer is a decidedly "choreophobic" gesture. Concerned about what turns a solo performer into a transgressive and/or out-of-control subject in solo improvisational Iranian dance, Shay coins the term "choreophobia" to mean "the negative and ambiguous reactions and feelings toward solo improvised dancing expressed by Iranians and other individuals and groups from the Middle East" (*Choreophobia* 7). Shay maintains that the performer draws known elements from "the enormous storehouse of variation" (46) in order to combine and create something fresh.

135

*Dora Stratou
and the
Construction
of Greek
Folklore*

Therefore, the dancer who performs in a way that signifies unpredictable, potentially out-of-control behaviour is likely to choose from a set vocabulary of movements stored in the tradition of that particular dance. If the Greek male dancer is playing with this sort of unpredictability, Stratou isn't. Dora Stratou refuses to take risks and resists the accreditation of the individual body with cultural production, fearing the transgression of recognizable and respectable boundaries by the solo dancer. Only the group is entitled to render tradition in a controlled choreography as censored by her. That a dancer's initiative and solo performance plays a significant part in Greek dance tradition is proven by Stratou's reference to it and subsequent attempt to assuage any fear that the dancer's "dionysiac" excess might inspire. It seems unlikely that she would be as perturbed if it were a minor, rare, or innocuous sign.

Stratou's insistence on control of a dancer's potential excesses still resonates throughout the Greek-speaking world. Her conservatism informs the conservatism of Greek communities especially outside Greece. Throughout my years in Canada, I have maintained an ambiguous relationship with the diasporic Greek and Greek-Cypriot communities. While I longed to be in their midst, speaking the language and engaging in the familiar customs and social activities that have bestowed upon me significant aspects of my identity, I also dreaded the strict conservatism and scrutiny to which I was subjected each time I sought participation. This precarious relationship took an interesting turn following my serious involvement with Oriental dance, an art form that, as I outline in this project, has come to assuage all the contraries of my ethnic and gender identity. Although the tsifteteli has not waned in popularity, it remains controversial and feared in its solo performance. The zeibekiko is also solo and largely improvised but assertively and aggressively masculine, while the kalamatiano is decidedly communal, thus offering a unique opportunity for bonding among the Greeks of the diaspora. When participating in a Greek party (γλέντι), the challenge for me as a solo dancer becomes how to interpret those bouzouki strains that spell out enthrallment in my ears, without exhibiting behaviour that is transgressive or "out of control." Shay's *Choreophobia* speaks to my anxieties and informs my questions about my participation in a critical, austere, and highly complex community with a remarkably long tradition.[9] Sadly, however, many times when I did decide to perform a bolder articulation of the moves, I realized that many of the participants feigned a nonchalant,

"I have seen
this dance on
old Greek
vases":
Hellenism
and the
Worlding of
Greek Dance

indifferent gaze to my choreography. This gaze is hardly characteristic of Greek sensibility in the context of a social event, where staring and gossiping are fairly popular as entertainment but also in regulating behaviour and managing social policing. Yet, nonchalance and indifference turn the male dancing body into a taboo, as in the case of Mousbah Baalbaki. As a form of condemnation, this indifferent gaze picks up from where Stratou ends her comment and concludes the sentence that she pronounces on othered embodiment and artistic interpretation. It signifies a gesture similar to what Stephen Murray terms "the will not to know" of homosexual behaviour, as if the lack of acknowledgement will make something vanish or deny its existence altogether. What Stratou contends in the choreophobic passage above has left a residual attitude of indifference and lack of acknowledgement. Ultimately, the purpose is to keep the hegemonic structure in place.

The Politics of Performance in "Greek" Cyprus

The Greek verb for producing yarn, *klotho*, has an interesting metaphorical application in the Cypriot dialect. In the island's cultural history, as I know it, the verb has been turned into an image that describes a particular kind of improper, suggestive movement. Someone who *klothetai*, or weaves her steps and moves the hips with sinuous motion, is one who indulges in an excessive, disagreeable performance of her femininity. The pejorative connotations are worse when the metaphor is used for a man. In his case, the verb would both deride his masculine performance and doubt his virility. The language of weaving to describe a disagreeable gender performance has obvious implications for both dance and discourse. Undulation of the midriff and waist are necessary articulations in the lexicon of Middle Eastern dance, yet in the popular imagination such choreographing of the body's narrative is a taboo. For example, that my gait might have a "weaving" quality to it was a constant nightmare during my adolescence. Movement is full of significations and, as Susan Foster indicates in "Choreographing History,"

> each body's movements all day long form part of the skeleton of meaning that also gives any aberrant or spectacular bodily action its luster. Those everyday patterns of movement make seduction or incarceration, hysteria or slaughter, routinization or recreation matter more distinctively. The writing body in the constant outpouring of its signification offers up nuances of meaning that make a difference. (5)

I have ventured into considerable detail regarding Stratou's discourse on Greek dances because it forms a lucid manifestation of the workings of power, a paradigm of nationalist forces setting the parameters of acceptable kinesthetic expression. This discourse also distills the principles that affected the pedagogy of my elementary school years in Cyprus in the early 1970s. The austerity and didacticism of her text resonated with official national policy. During our physical education class we were taught some of those dances that Stratou established as "panhellenic": the kalamatianos, syrtos, and tsamikos (although the onus for learning the dances in my school was on the girls rather than the boys since dancing was deemed more fitting for girls). Lisbet Torp, in her article "'It's All Greek to Me': The Invention of Pan-Hellenic Dances—and Other Stories," discusses the kalamatiano and tsamiko as dances that originated in the areas liberated after the Greek War of Independence of 1821, and were systematically taught in the main towns of the newly formed Greek state. These dances thus came to symbolize a newly freed Greece. The other important connection with my argument here is that the Greek War of Independence was decided at the naval battle of Lepanto where French, British, and German ships defeated the Ottoman fleet. This victory by Western colonial powers determined their involvement in the character as well as administration of the new Greek state.

On the national front, through its time as a republic, Cyprus has been overcome by an unrelenting Islamophobia. This outlook has accommodated hatred, as well as fear deriving from a constant threat of violence and devastation on all levels—territorial, national, and bodily (manifest in the fear of rape). Complicating these fears, while also perpetuating them, was the validation of a European attitude that Edward Said outlines as follows:

> Not for nothing did Islam come to symbolize terror, devastation, the demonic, hordes of hated barbarians. For Europe, Islam was a lasting trauma. Until the end of the seventeenth century the "Ottoman peril" lurked alongside Europe to represent for the whole of Christian civilization a constant danger, and in time European civilization incorporated that peril and its lore, its great events, figures, virtues, and vices, as something woven into the fabric of life. (*Orientalism* 59-60)

The fall of Byzantium to the Ottomans in 1453 is one of the traumas that have become lore in the Greek imagination. This loss has been endlessly mourned and narrated. It is regarded as "cultural contamination analogous to the consequences for humanity at large of original sin"

"I have seen
this dance on
old Greek
vases":
Hellenism
and the
Worlding of
Greek Dance

(Herzfeld, "Hellenism and Orientalism" 219). Apparently, though, the Islamic menace was a wider and more pervasive concern manifest on many different occasions. At the Centennial Exhibition of 1876 in Philadelphia, the Turkish exhibition received particularly telling reviews in the *New York Daily Tribune*:

> There is a natural anxiety to find out what is made by the strange Asiatic people who have possessed for more than four centuries the fairest part of Europe, driving out the Christian religion from its early strongholds and defying the fundamental ideas of European civilization. (qtd. in Monty 18)

It was easy for European influence, exerted during the colonial occupation, to transmit to Cyprus the symbolic significations that Said has theorized. Following British rule, any effects of colonialism were largely ignored by the newly born republic in the face of fear and loathing for the infidel Turk, who came to dominate the thought and action of the Greek-Cypriot people as the sole enemy of the new nation. As Benedict Anderson argues, the term "republic" itself is national and grounds itself "firmly in a territorial and social space inherited from the prerevolutionary past" (2).[10] Belly dance as cultural phenomenon and as artistic expression hardly achieved the status of anything more than a derided Eastern, that is, Turkish, cultural institution. Because of Islam's traumatic impact on Greek Cyprus, the dance was further condemned to unspeakability, shrouded with the taboo of silence. Parallel to this propaganda that forfeited Eastern signs, elements of Greek culture were suppressed, a movement accounting for the objections to the Greek entry at the Eurovision Song Contest of 1976; a "consent from below." (As I discuss in chapter 1, the issues arising from this event signalled a critical moment for my subjectivity—a moment when I was forced to choose my allegiances and I was prepared, and quite eager I now realize, to love both extravagantly: belly dance and Mariza.)

In their schooling, young students were taught to adopt a subjectivity whose parameters were dictated by Western ideologies.[11] Studying folk songs (Δημοτικά Τραγούδια) of Greece at high school, we giggled as we came across descriptions of strapping youthful men described in the songs as having a lithe waist and a swaying gait. I had to laugh along so as not to exacerbate the already injurious gap that separated me from my peers. Yet I was enamoured of the image of a man in this particular embodiment of masculinity, a romanticized image that I found a great deal more appealing than the butch, macho stereotype of my day. Appar-

139

*The Tsifteteli,
Grecian
Orientalism,
and the Male
Dancer*

ently, in the tradition of various Greek regions, this swaying that we laughed at because it seemed—anachronistically—"gay" to our puerile, colonially inflected minds, was a particular way of gesturing that celebrated youth, health, beauty, and artistic talent, an attribute that was essential in the conception of valour in folk constructions of male behaviour. Our giggles confirmed that artistic talent had lost most of its currency and that we were all genuine children of technology and heterosexual virility (I was never, of course, convincing in any of these roles).

Most significantly for us in the present, the movement described in Greek folk songs is one that predates European colonization in the region. In 1961, Nearhos Clerides asserts (with that patronizing confidence that hegemonic ideology endows a speaker) that Cypriot women's folk dances (and he is clearly implying Greek Cypriot) derive from a traditional Greek fairy tale, while bravery and valour characterize the men's dances whose main purpose is "to incite the admiration and respect of the audience, particularly the fair sex"! And he continues:

> The dancers' posture is firm and upright, the gaze and the movements rhythmical. The folding or the bending of the legs, lowering the head, and any movements of the waist are entirely foreign to the authentic Cypriot dances and are, instead, characteristics of corresponding Turkish men's dances. (4, my translation)

Clerides's construction of Cypriot dance is rife with sexism and racism. He completely disregards Turkish Cypriot dance traditions and relies for his analysis on the assumption that "Cypriot" (Greek) artistic expression has nothing in common with the Turkish community of the island or with its neighbouring Middle Eastern cultures. He also proceeds to justify the Turkish term *karçilama* that Greek Cypriots use for a set of male and female dances and concludes that the Turkish term better expresses the character of the dance as involving a meeting of sorts and not just a performance. Clerides's arguments are obviously unconvincing and contradictory, yet the discourse that he developed had great currency in the young republic.

The Tsifteteli, Grecian Orientalism, and the Male Dancer

Of course, Dora Stratou's discourse on Greek dances did not eradicate the tsifteteli or those elements in Greek music and dance that were deemed "Eastern" and therefore undesirable. As Gail Holst-Warhaft points out, "despite the successful propagation of the myth of cultural

"I have seen
this dance on
old Greek
vases":
Hellenism
and the
Worlding of
Greek Dance

continuity, Greeks continued to insist on a model of community-based affiliation that was often at variance with official ideology and frequently crossed linguistic and ethnic boundaries" ("Song, Self-Identity and the Neohellenic" 232). Using the examples of left-wing opposition and its production of music as resistance from the early 1950s to the mid-1960s, the Pontic Greeks who perform to music indistinguishable from that of their Turkish counterparts, and the Rebetes who defy societal norms, Holst-Warhaft exposes the phenomenon of Greeks embracing their national identity, while also defining themselves through song as inhabitants of a subgroup that transgresses in some respects, the boundaries and/or ideals of the state (232-33).

Especially the Pontic Greeks' dances present a unique example of a tradition that has preserved a dance vocabulary quite unlike that of any other Greek region. They accompany their dances with their indigenous type of rebec and daoul (a large drum similar to the Egyptian doholla). However, a significant Pontic dance move that is not encountered in the dances of any other Greek region today is the shoulder shimmy. This is a move that has been an important part of Middle Eastern dance expression, the same move that Kuchuk Hanem and Azizeh performed for the khawadjas (Azizeh has been described shimmying the shoulders as well; I discuss her moves in chapter 4). Due to the relative remoteness of their geographical location, the Pontic peoples remained apart from the rest of Greek populations during the formative years of Greek nationhood. This isolation might account for the unique vocabularies their dances display. They remained unaffected by the discourse of Occidentalism that persuaded those individuals who claimed authority in transcribing traditions. These included dancers and dance instructors (such as those working for the Dora Stratou theatre, but also others working independently) who quite quickly became experts in all dances and disseminated an often arbitrary version of tradition to fulfill agendas of social, cultural, and ultimately state politics, thus perpetuating what they perceived as the "proper" versions of vernacular dances. That the shimmy survived only, as far as I know, in the dances of the Pontic Greeks tempts me to speculate on its possible existence in a range of Greek dances and its recent intentional elimination. It is a difficult move that not only requires skill but also signifies extremes, and a certain intensity that might be discomforting. Andrea Deagon finds the shimmy to be "a kind of motion that escapes, temporarily, countable time ... a trembling that represents extremes" ("Dance, Body, Universe" 17). I hear shimmying in many tra-

141

*The Tsifteteli,
Grecian
Orientalism,
and the Male
Dancer*

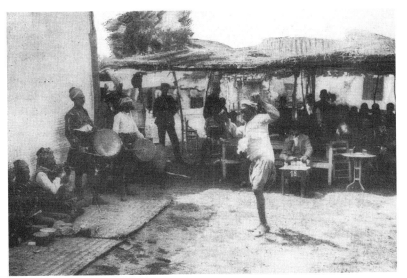

"Odemich, Turkish Dance." 1921. With the Greek army advancing into Asia Minor, cards are printed with landscapes and scenes from the new areas. This card depicts a Turkish man in local costume dancing at an outdoor coffee house. The musical instruments are two large drums (doholla), two zorna and small drums. (Comments by Alkis Raftis. My translation. Reprinted with permission from *Dance 1900: Greek Turn-of-the-Century Postcards Portraying Dance* by Alkis Raftis.)

ditional Greek songs so I am reluctant to accept that the shimmy has never formed part of any one of the different traditions that Stratou represented on the national and international stages. It denotes a "dionysiac" mood, an excited climax—precisely what she censures and tries to silence.

Stratou's project was given further urgency by historical developments that came to bear on the Greek cultural scene and which reassert the significance of the politics of music and dance. In 1922, huge populations from Asia Minor came to settle in Greece following their forced massive exodus from their towns on the Ionian coast. Their forced migration was the result of a tragic political development so disastrous for Greece that in the Greek world it is simply referred to as "The Catastrophe" [Η Καταστροφή]. Thousands of Christian, Greek-speaking people from the western coast of Asia Minor became the victims who paid the price for Greek attempts at imperialist expansion. The "Grand Idea" [Μεγάλη Ιδέα], as it is known, is "the doctrine of Greek irredentism whereby all the lands of Classical and Byzantine Hellenism should be reclaimed for the reborn nation" (Herzfeld, *Ours Once More* 119). To implement this "Grand Idea," an actual military landing took place on the

"I have seen
this dance on
old Greek
vases":
Hellenism
and the
Worlding of
Greek Dance

coast of Asia Minor in 1922, an operation that failed dismally and whose consequences were devastating both for Greece and the Christian, Greek-speaking populations of the Ionian coast. Their subsequent expulsion from the region became "enshrined in Greek popular culture as a metaphor for loss and grief" (Holst-Warhaft, "Rebetika" 115).

From a colonial discourse point of view, what I find most noteworthy in this dire historical development is the manner in which the Greek aspiration predicated itself on the model of an East-West conflict with Greece being, of course, on the West side of the binary. The "Grand Idea" was not an inherently Greek invention but the expression of expansionist politics shared by major colonial powers. It was, in other words, "part and parcel of colonialist logic" as Gourgouris puts it (146). Pursuing the vision of a sovereign Greece ruling over the lands that once included the Byzantine Empire demonstrates modern Greece's imperial aspirations. Following the ultimate failure of the expedition, a failure facilitated by the major European powers (Gourgouris 146-47), the people who flocked to Greece as refugees came to be regarded as a loathsome reminder of this failure and the nation's unwanted responsibility towards them. By extension, their cultural inheritance was regarded with a suspicion that graduated to persecution soon after they set up their first entertainment establishments on the Greek mainland.

The course that events took, however, forced Greece to confront these traditions that it found impossible to accept and incorporate. Following the Catastrophe, many of these victims left for Greece without their material possessions and arrived there destitute. Or rather, they were destitute except that many brought with them a musical heritage and an artistic sophistication that were rare in the Greek mainland. The urban centres of Constantinople and Smyrna were viable contact zones with artistic exchanges taking place constantly, more so in the areas of music and dance that were especially flourishing. These two places "were musically sophisticated towns where Turkish, Greek, Jewish, Armenian and Gypsy musicians played together and exchanged repertoires" (Holst-Warhaft, "Rebetika" 115). Unfortunately, the Greek establishment was unable to recognize the talent and artistic sophistication of these musical forms that came from Asia Minor, since their decidedly "Eastern" character provoked suspicion and disdain. Although loved and appreciated by many Greeks, it proved impossible for these musical traditions to influence official national policy as favourably as Stratou's projects managed to do in the 1960s. The refugees' music, that came to be known as "rebetika,"

143

*The Tsifteteli,
Grecian
Orientalism,
and the Male
Dancer*

was too strident to assimilate into the social homogeneity that modern Greece aspired towards. Rebetika simply could not qualify as native past or present and could not reflect an acceptable notion of national identity.

During the Metaxas dictatorship (1936–1940), musicians and singers who belonged to rebetika groups were harassed and many even exiled to the islands or imprisoned. Such drastic action was by no means arduous to undertake. The rebetes were not simply poor, working-class people who were often a target in the eyes of the law; many of them were already ex-convicts and/or hashish addicts frequenting hashish dens in Piraeus. Metaxas shut down many of these establishments, not merely because they were disreputable, but, as Gail Holst-Warhaft points out, because they disrupted Metaxas's vision of a reified "Third Hellenic Civilization," consciously based on Hitler's Third Reich ("World Music and the Orientalising of the Rebetika"). This ambitious accomplishment would draw its character from "appropriate" reconstructions of Greek folkloric culture—not from a musical legacy direct from Asia Minor. In this climate of refashioning and censorship, *amanedhes* (singular *amanes*), a characteristically Eastern mode of singing, also underwent scrutiny and, eventually, ban. These were (still are) a type of vocal improvisation that often becomes the showpiece for the singer's musical talents and sophistication. They are profoundly emotional vocal passages where pathos and grief are expressed through both the lyrics and the dirge-like quality of the singing. Holst-Warhaft suggests that *amanedhes* were banned during Metaxas's dictatorship, "probably as a response to a similar ban placed on them by Turkey's ruler, Kemal Ataturk. Ataturk's ban was part of a general attempt to westernize Turkey, and de-emphasize its "oriental" character" ("World Music and the Orientalising of the Rebetika").[12]

Apart from *amandhes*, the rebetiko repertoire included mainly the solo improvisational dances of the zeibekiko and the tsifteteli and a pair or group dance, the hasapiko. Rebetes, their music, and their establishments (often wooden huts or cottages) were severely censured by the authorities because of a combination of factors that I believe bears an intricate connection to issues emerging from the ideology of Greek identity. The Rebetes' society saw itself as independent, and its identity was partly based on a common mistrust of the rest of Greek society. In the words of Gail Holst-Warhaft, their music was "the creative expression of their independence." Holst-Warhaft locates the appeal of rebetika in the *taksim* (the opening passage that introduces the *makam*, or musical road, of the piece that follows), the lyrics, and the dance.[13] These artistic com-

"I have seen
this dance on
old Greek
vases":
Hellenism
and the
Worlding of
Greek Dance

ponents "are still close to the magic of spontaneous creativity, and yet they have the surety of a tradition behind them, and a social framework where musician and listener are united by the mutual recognition of being outside, and in many respects superior to the rest of society" (*Road to Rembetika* 77).

Rebetika attributes were not what the Dora Stratou tradition would respect, appreciate, or even approve of. In her attempts to reinvent Greek dance, the "surety of a tradition" that Holst-Warhaft identifies as part of the rebetika would be anathema. With her strong, right-wing connections, Stratou denied not only the artistic and cultural value of rebetika but also any connection between tsifteteli and classical Greek dances, in a gesture that complies with the construction of Western civilization as the heritage of classical Greece. In Greece, therefore, the tsifteteli gradually came to be marginalized—banned into the region of undesirable, distasteful influences of the Orient.

Ironically, these attempts to sacrifice the tsifteteli on the altar of classical glamour confirmed not only its survival but also its influence. Compelled to contend with its signification, some dance enthusiasts did not adhere to Stratou's total silencing of this art. Their attempts to retrieve it, however, involved similar ideological constructs. For example, the German scholar Ulf Buchheld undertook meticulous research to confirm the ancient Greek roots of the tsifteteli. He identifies it as a dance with a clearly erotic character and this, he believes, disqualifies it as a dance of ancient Greek tragedy (36). Buchheld's scholarship is broad, meticulous, and well documented, yet he still discourses within the parameters of sexism and gender discrimination. His prejudice is evident in the following comment that is an eerie echo of Özdemir's conviction of what belly dance means: "Mainly and justifiably [the tsifteteli] is danced by women, since the shimmying of the breasts, the gyration of the hips, and the swaying of the body *find their meaning only in the arousal of the man*" (my emphasis, my translation, 36)!

A less blatantly sexist but still problematic "recuperation" of the tsifteteli is undertaken by Theodore and Elfleida Petrides in their book *Folk Dances of the Greeks*. Theirs is one of those remote attempts to assign a purportedly classical connection to the tsifteteli and thus situate it in the pantheon of Greek dance (59-61). The Petrides trace the origins of the tsifteteli (which they call "kelikos horos," a literal translation of "danse du ventre") to the ancient worship of Mother Earth and Aphrodite (whom they call "Moon Goddess"). They interpret its undulating movements as

145

The Tsifteteli,
Grecian
Orientalism,
and the Male
Dancer

a depiction of the serpent and water, both representing symbols of the Moon Goddess. They state confidently that its ancient Greek name was "kolia" and that, following the fall of Byzantium, the dance was denigrated by the Arab and Turkish conquerors! The Petrides bypass rebetika completely and offer an explanation that relies on a historical assumption that conflates romanticist notions with nationalist concerns.[14]

This imperialist discourse has been successful in perpetuating a kind of homelessness. That is, a large range of subjects and their circumstances qualify for the trope of homelessness: the refugee from Smyrna who sings in Turkish and hums Eastern maqams to herself, the average Greek schoolboy in Thessaloniki who is taught aversion towards his "gypsy" and Muslim classmates, the Greek-speaking Cypriot who turns from traditions with derision since they signify an undesirable lineage. This homelessness also qualifies as a sexual homelessness since the politics of gender, class, sexuality, race, and ethnos are inextricably woven into the social body of the polis as well as the individual body. Avenues of cultural expression that close correspond to avenues of sexual fulfillment that are blocked by heterosexual orthodoxy.

In the article that I refer to at the opening of this chapter, Angela Shand configures identity, theology, and gender as the three agents that have been formative in the reception of this dance in modern Greece. She explains that each of these agents empowers ideological strategies as it diminishes every aspect of the dance that could be deemed attractive. The fact that the tsifteteli has been designated as feminine expression in the dynamic of a paternalistic society has extinguished any possibility that this dance could express something other than common female seduction and an invitation to sin. Ulf Buchheld's take on the tsifteteli certainly extinguishes such possibilities, especially when he concludes that this dance is rooted deeply in Greek antiquity but did not have a part in tragedy since it was confined to an expression of eroticism mainly portrayed by women. (Of course, women did not participate in performances of ancient Greek plays but Buchheld does not dwell extensively on this subject.) These conclusions are by no means radical or even innovative. They merely bolster the patriarchal order of dance procedures perpetuating the same limiting views just as the scholar, Buchheld, challenges the embarrassed silence on the tsifteteli in the Greek cultural context and believes himself to be reinstating it as a Greek dance.

In an otherwise poorly written article entitled "I Remember Nadia," Suhaila Salimpur, perhaps inadvertently, opens up a dimension of the

"I have seen
this dance on
old Greek
vases":
Hellenism
and the
Worlding of
Greek Dance

dance that liberates the dancer from this male-induced political order. While she narrates her childhood encounter with Nadia Gamal, a Lebanese dancer of great talent and fame, Salimpur records an anecdotal dialogue between her and the dancer. Their exchange is significant for the kinesthetic philosophy it relays:

"Do you know why I dance the way I do?" [Nadia Gamal] asked me. "Because I have suffered. I have gone through divorce, death, a lot of heartache ... that's the art. You can show anyone a step, but not a soul." I said I would go home and work on suffering right away. She told me never to forget why I dance. It would always give me strength. And she told me to "always remember the music."

Indeed, rebetika songs performed to the tsifteteli rhythm often thematize emotions of pain, heartache, and suffering. The contemporary approach that wants to confine this dance to an exuberant expression of joy, or more commonly, female seductive charm and sexual playfulness or coyness cannot be taken as absolute and needs to be challenged.[15] In fact, to see the tsifteteli as merely an expression of happiness (which is by no means a negative attribute—of course) denotes an attempt to trivialize it by limiting its possibility for expression of other human emotions considered to be profound or great. Tahia Carioca, the revered Egyptian dancer, feels that dignity is the most important quality in a dancer, yet, also, the dancer "must express life, death, happiness, sorrow, love and anger" (qtd. in Monty 306).

This contemplative, introspective character of the tsifteteli, which is audible in old rebetika, has not survived very well. In the process of cultural selection, other dances whose popularity in Asia Minor was also great, such as the zeibekiko and the hasapiko, gained extremely high cultural currency since they were perceived as harmonious with, in fact enhancing, the popular construction of masculine behaviour. Contemplation and introspection have been saved for the zeibekiko, in particular, which symbolizes the male ethos and enjoys widespread recognition as the expression of an indomitable masculinity, a respected and valued disposition. Its steps reify a certain machismo that has been normalized and expected of a man. The zeibekiko inscribes territorial boundaries that the viewer observes with comfort, but also awe and admiration since it ritualizes an exemplary masculinity and evokes the desire in the viewer to approve and emulate. Describing how the zeibekiko is performed, Elias Petropoulos goes into rapture:

147

*The Tsifteteli,
Grecian
Orientalism,
and the Male
Dancer*

*Αφού ο ζεϊμπέκικος δεν έχει τυποποιημένο βηματισμό οι φιγούρες αποκτούν
εξέχουσα θέση. Ο ζεϊμπέκικος φωτίζει τον χορευτή, τον κάνει ωραίο σαν
μικρό θεό. Χορεύεται ο ζεϊμπέκικος ίσα κι ίσα, με χέρια και με πόδια. Ο
σπαθάτος χορευτής του ζεϊμπέκικου, στεγνός, με πεσμένο στούς γοφούς παν —
τελόνι, κάνει μια σειρά από θεσπέσια παραπατήματα σαν δέντρο που
σείεται.... Ο ζεϊμπέκικος χορεύεται με τα χέρια σε στάση δεήσως, ή ικεσίας.*
(38)

Since the zeibekiko does not have a typical choreography, the moves
acquire a special significance. The zeibekiko illuminates the dancer, beau-
tifies him like a miniature god. The zeibekiko is performed with both arms
and feet used equally. The zeibekiko dancer, lithe and slender, with his
pants loose on his hips, performs a series of splendid false steps like a swaying tree.... Zeibekiko is danced with the hands in the position of prayer
or supplication. (My translation 38)

The contrast with the solo dancer about to exhibit transgressive behaviour and the choreophobia he inspires is quite striking and brings the
performance of gender and sexuality in dance into sharp relief. Nonetheless, this ritualization of masculinity is also invested with a strongly queer
quality. In the homoerotic gaze of Greek artists such as the painter Yian-
nis Tsarouhis and the composer Manos Hadjidakis, the attraction of this
masculine expression was undeniably compelling.[16] The masculinity performed in the zeibekiko is so exalted that even if the dancer transgresses
during improvisation he is still guaranteed acceptance.[17] Moreover, the
devotion to this dance is so strong that even though the zeibekiko can
be traced to Asia Minor, there is no anxiety to justify its existence in the
Greek dance repertoire. Conversely, such anxiety determines the discourse around the tsifteteli whose "origins" in the East are invoked repeatedly.[18] Thus the dance and its movements have become established as a
signifier of the East and of unbridled female sexuality.

Even Gail Holst-Warhaft, who is an accomplished scholar of modern
Greek culture (particularly music and dance traditions), proceeds to make
problematic and somewhat carelessly presented statements regarding this
dance's performance. While discussing the male homosocial world of the
Rebetes, she makes certain observations which I find disconcerting:

This is a world that not only excludes women, but celebrates their absence.
Interestingly, even the one dance of the rebetika repertoire that was essentially a woman's dance, the tsifte-teli, was not uncommonly performed
by men holding their genitals as they gyrated in a lewd parody of female
dancing. ("Rebetika: The Double Descended Deep Songs of Greece" 121)

I object to Holst-Warhaft's comments for several reasons. She does not cite the context she refers to, thus encouraging the reader to speculate on the origins of such information: is this a moment of personal witness (rather unlikely since Holst-Warhaft is female and the setting here is very male), or did an informant supply the information? By being vague, Holst-Warhaft affords the phenomenon she describes an overwhelming reach, thus harming the reputation of the dance. Furthermore, by relating information of this kind, she vulgarizes the tsifteteli since she focuses attention on particularly distasteful performances of a dance that already suffers because of poor representations. Finally, despite her great interest in the historical roots of rebetika, her artistic participation in Greek musical groups in the 1970s, and all the valuable research she has conducted on the subject, Holst-Warhaft accepts without questioning that the tsifteteli is an "essentially women's dance." By reiterating such statements from uncited sources, Holst-Warhaft perpetuates the distorted notions of this dance and even re-presents its male performers as engrossed in misogynist parody.[19]

To demonstrate the spurious nature of Holst-Warhaft's representation, I refer to an episode from a documentary musical series on Greek television entitled "Our Old Friends" ("Οι Παλιοί μας Φίλοι"). The series was filmed in the early 1980s and was dedicated to the older generation of Greek singers and songwriters, many of them famous exponents of the rebetika tradition. In the opening scene of the episode depicting the life and career of Yiota Lydia, the viewer is introduced to two young teenage boys who ride a motorcycle wearing headphones and listening to an old tsifteteli by Lydia. As they park their vehicle outside a building, their attention is drawn by music and loud conversation. The two young men proceed to gaze voyeuristically through the window of an all-male coffee shop at a moustached soldier in uniform performing tsifteteli.[20] The scene depicts nothing suggestive of lewdness or misogynist parody in the soldier's choreography. He shimmies the shoulders which he also uses to pronounce the accents in the song, and then proceeds in an exhibition of physical strength—and machismo by extension—by performing various feats, all to the counts of the music. His colleagues (many of the men present are also in army uniform) manifest their approval by clapping and shouting words of encouragement. The air in the room is thick with cigarette smoke, exaltation, and feelings of admiration for the dancer. He concludes his performance by dancing towards a chair, lifting it with his teeth, and holding it up in the air as he performs the final steps of the

149

The Tsifteteli,
Grecian
Orientalism,
and the Male
Dancer

song's ending. If his demonstrations of physical strength help to diffuse the compelling homoerotic energy of the scene, they also, paradoxically, build it further.

This dance scene is one of those rare filmic moments that so spontaneously make the male dancing body the subject of voyeuristic indulgence. The soldier is enjoyed by his colleagues, by the younger men who watch through the window (the glass separates them as a barrier but also enhances the magic of the moment), and by the TV audience that is also "looking" through the camera as it films the boys. It is pleasing that different generations of males are introduced to the eloquence and imaginative potential of this scene. Moreover, the involvement of the young teenage spectators is a tender moment of male socialization in an intensely homoerotic environment, a rite of passage of sorts, rendered all the more poignant by equivocal signifiers of desire. I credit Yiorgos Papastefanou, a sensitive and well-informed lover and critic of Greek music and dance, as the inspired creator of this rare scenario that introduces this particular episode. While the soldier dances, Papastefanou is heard describing briefly the tsifteteli. In the description he quotes the opening sentence from the following audaciously sexist passage on the tsifteteli from Elias Petropoulos's *Rebetika*:

Το τσιφτετέλι θέλει κεφάτο σείσιμο του στήθους και κάποιον αισθησιασμό στίς κινήσεις τής μέσης καί τών γοφών . Οι γυναίκες με τα τρεμουλιαστά βυζιά, τους παχουλούς γλουτούς και το γλυκό χαμόγελο χορεύουν το τσιφτετέλι με ασυγκρίτως μεγαλύτερην επιτυχίαν απο τους άντρες. Μάλιστα συχνά το τσιφτετέλι χορεύεται πάνω σε τραπέζι γεμάτο πιατικά (τότε είναι σωστή αποθέωση του γυναικείου κορμιού), για να μην μπορεί η χορεύτρια να κάνει βήματα, παρά μόνο να λυγίζει το σώμα, ενώ κάτω η παρέα της χτυπάει παλαμάκια.

The tsifteteli requires vivacious shimmying of the chest and a certain sensuality in the movement of the waist and the hips. Women with quivering breasts, plump thighs, and sweet smile dance the tsifteteli with a level of success incomparable to that of men. In fact, the tsifteteli is often performed on a table covered with dishes (then it is the real apotheosis of the female body), so that the dancer cannot take steps except sway her body, while her friends below clap. (My translation, 39)

Through this reading at this particular moment, Papastefanou deconstructs Petropoulos' comments that this dance is performed by women "with a level of success incomparable to that of men" (notably, Petropoulos assumes that men do perform this dance as well), and further problematizes Holst-Warhaft's remarks on the lewd, parodied renditions of

"I have seen
this dance on
old Greek
vases":
Hellenism
and the
Worlding of
Greek Dance

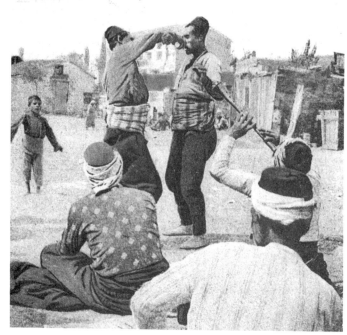

"Salonica—the Belly Dance." 1916-1917. Muslim men perform belly dance somewhere in Macedonia. (Comments by Alkis Raftis. My translation. Reprinted with permission from *Dance 1900: Greek Turn-of-the-Century Postcards Portraying Dance* by Alkis Raftis.)

the tsifteteli. As the moustached soldier crosses his arms across his chest and makes his lower body vibrate in an intense shimmy, Petropoulos's sexist affirmations resonate jarringly.

That men do not have the "right" figure and are neither graceful nor "attractive" enough to perform Middle Eastern dance seems a popular sexist misconception. In the PBS documentary series *Dancing*, based on Gerald Jonas's book by the same title, the Moroccan sociologist Mohammad Chtatou comments (in English) that dance is "womanly, not manly," thus supporting Jonas's comment that "there is no masculine equivalent to the dance that Muslim women practice" (115). Moreover, if male spectators join the public dancers they will "undulate their shoulders and hips in what looks like a self-mocking parody of traditional gender roles, combined with sheer delight in rhythmic physical movement" (116). That Jonas's comments echo Holst-Warhaft's is an indication that such views are not simply the result of superficial observations but the work of ideology. In a critique of both Jonas's remarks and the cor-

151

*The Tsifteteli,
Grecian
Orientalism,
and the Male
Dancer*

responding scene from the documentary, Anthony Shay points out that "Jonas should have at least been suspicious that his statements were misleading because the footage accompanying Chtatou's questionable observations, heard in a voiceover, showed a large group of men dancing with great enjoyment, the very dancing he describes as female" ("The Male Dancer" 16-17).

At the conclusion of the film *Satin Rouge* there is a similar dance moment where the male performer is pushed to the margins despite his contribution of dancing and singing that imbue the entire scene with a magnificent sensuality. This is the final movie scene of the wedding party of Lilia's daughter. As the guest singer performs at the party, his singing emanates not only from his throat. His entire body is melodious as he moves across the scene, interacting with Lilia and her guests, all the while articulating the music with great charisma. Moreover, the eloquence, flair, and flamboyance that mark his masculine embodiment provide a refreshing change from the heterosexism of the men who gaze at the female dancers in the cabaret scenes of the film (even though a number of them move fluently to the rhythms of the darabukeh, the hand drum).[21] However, this male singer's performance is not highlighted the way Lilia's is. Her dance technique is poor throughout, but in this scene her dancing is particularly awkward with her arms impeding her kinesthetic expression instead of enhancing or even assisting it. She is dancing before her son-in-law whom she had had a sexual affair with just before the wedding, and next to a male singer and dancer whose sexual and sensual embodiment are distinctly poignant; understandably, perhaps, her performance is awkward. Her male friend and colleague (he is also her hairdresser) who sings and dances for the guests comes across as someone whose part is taken for granted, and, even though his role at the party is central, he is portrayed as an artist who frames the scene rather than being at the heart of it. He is also used as an agent that deflates some of the tension between Lilia and Chokri, the groom (her ex-lover and now son-in-law). The performer's grace and talent are not showcased for their great artistic value, while his distinct embodiment of masculinity and charm are left to the perception of inquisitive viewers who search for meanings in marginal and disused spaces.

While traversing the gender and sexuality divide, I am conscious of the politics of nation playing their significant part. Located on the cusp of these politics, Roza Eskenazy, a singer and dancer and one of the most attractive and beloved "rebetisses," constitutes simultaneously an inter-

"I have seen
this dance on
old Greek
vases":
Hellenism
and the
Worlding of
Greek Dance

esting embodiment of "Greekness" and alterity. She was a Jewish-Greek-Armenian artist originally from Constantinople—a lineage that makes her a veritable meeting point of cultures from the Middle East. When she was first approached by Panayiotis Toundas, a popular songwriter interested in recording with her, she felt dismayed because he asked her to sing "kalamatiano" on a record. "What is a kalamatiano, I asked them—I know of no such thing; this is the first time I hear it!" (My translation, Eskenazy 20). I am intrigued to contemplate the meaning of Roza's

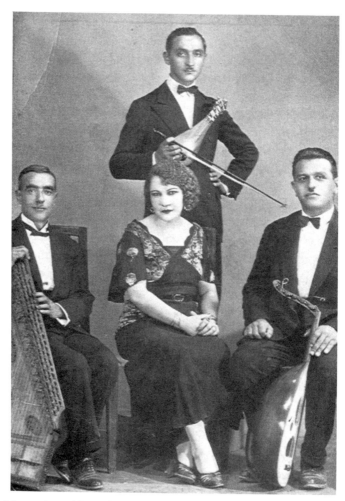

Roza Eskenazy in a publicity photo with her musicians: Lambros Liondaridies on the rebec (centre), Agapios Tomboulis on the oud (right), an unidentified qanoon player on the left. Circa 1936 (Elias Petropoulos, *Rebetika Tragoudia*)

153

*The Tsifteteli,
Grecian
Orientalism,
and the Male
Dancer*

"Greekness" as I imagine her on a humble wooden stage performing Turkish and Greek songs to the sound of the qanoon and the violin, dancing and keeping the rhythm with her finger cymbals—a performance that is radically different from Stratou's spectacular renditions of Greek classical tradition. When Eskenazy began her career in rebetika groups in the 1930s as a singer and dancer, she hardly knew Greek and was also unfamiliar with the bouzouki, the instrument that the film *Zorba the Greek* would soon establish as the most prevalent and widely marketed signifier of "Greekness."[22] Santoor, qanoon, violin, and guitar were the instruments she would sing to. In fact, she confesses to not being too fond of the bouzouki at first. Of course, in her subsequent recording career, this instrument was ubiquitous, including her tsifteteli songs. Yet even later in her life (I remember her on black-and-white TV in the late 1970s), she retained her alterity, appearing in harem pants and embroidered vests—apparel that appealed to me greatly and created a lasting memory.

With the tsifteteli, its exponents, its audience, and its performers in Greece, I contend that the issue moved beyond the identity of a subgroup. Since the appeal of this dance could not be eradicated, hegemony concentrated its efforts on denigrating its social status, and therefore influence, by relegating it to a class phenomenon instead. In fact, the tsifteteli became necessary in defining "civilization" and class. Lower working classes were, in a sense, assigned their own music known in popular language as folk urban music (Λαϊκή μουσική).[23] Especially the kind that featured "coarse and uncomely" Eastern strains that lacked the refinement of Western music, (which Dora Stratou learned to sing to and play on the piano as a child) gradually became the expression of low-income and largely uneducated wage earners who lived in the villages or in the underprivileged quarters of the rapidly sprawling urban centres of Thessaloniki and Athens. Refugees from the Ionian coast settled in both cities but it was especially in Piraeus and Thessaloniki that the rebetika culture was the strongest in numbers and influence. Stelios Kazantzides, a Pontic Greek, and Yiota Lydia, herself a refugee from Smyrna, became two of the most popular voices of tsifteteli songs. Both singers introduced a new quality into Greek urban folk songs that appealed to a new generation of working-class Greeks.[24] Conversely, moneyed and therefore refined and educated Greeks persevered in their role as guardians of the classical traditions and Greece's Western character. They attended Stratou's performances but also entertained themselves with European dances such as the waltz, the foxtrot, as well as other dances, the tango and the

"I have seen
this dance on
old Greek
vases":
Hellenism
and the
Worlding of
Greek Dance

rumba being among them. These may not be Western dances in derivation but were imported from the West and therefore signified a certain
refinement and cosmopolitanism. In this way, relegating the tsifteteli to
an inferior class status has been a means of controlling it but also preserving it in a circumspect order as opposed to discarding it completely. This
politic enacts the interlocking of desire and derision in a hegemonic operation to sustain what is desirable but control its contagion.

Including Greece and the politics of the tsifteteli in this project does
not rely entirely on the enactment of Orientalist politics within the Hellenic context, or on the fact that certain Egyptian rhythms form the foundation of many popular Greek songs.[25] The inclusion itself implies a
political decision. As I point out in the introduction to this chapter, the
Orient is a formidable signifier in the Greek imaginary. Even so, there
are Greeks who accept being perpetually situated in the interstices of
East and West. What is problematic—and perhaps irresolvable—about
such assertions is that the very existence of this in-between location is
sanctioned by the dominant imperial discourse of colonialist Europe and
becomes, by extension, yet another manifestation of its power. Claims
from the country itself about its situation between East and West have
become cliché in modern travel discourse. Apart from Greece and Cyprus,
I have read and heard of similar claims made about places as geographically disparate as Iran, Egypt, Morocco, and Turkey. What I find most significant is that travel documentaries or literature are not the only sites
that offer such locations. Often the countries themselves will adopt the
crossroads motif as essential in their self-description and, by extension,
self-definition. At times, this position is even a matter of national pride.
What worries me is the issue of compromise in this positioning and its concomitant anxiety in a postcolonial state of affairs. At times, I hear it as
an apology to the West: an apology for the minarets, the adobe villages,
the extended-family system. Often it is stated in the hope that it will
relieve the exigencies and pressures of inhabiting an ambivalent location. In the case of Greece, the interesting fact is that its self-positioning
falls within familiar colonialist tropes even though it has never been colonized administratively.

As I conclude this chapter, I would like to revisit certain terms that
merit further explication. Alkis Raftis, the board president of the Dora
Stratou Theatre, calls Stratou's contribution a "living museum," a term
intended to commend the scope and accomplishment of the foundation
(Shay, Choreographic Politics 267). Yet, in this postcolonial state of affairs,

155

*The Tsifteteli,
Grecian
Orientalism,
and the Male
Dancer*

I have to ponder the ideological implications of such characterization. As Inderpal Grewal asserts, in a metropolitan setting, "the museum displayed realms of knowledge that had earlier been hidden from the general public and provided the proximity of valuable objects that without any possibility of possession aroused the pride of national ownership" (125). The "valuable object" in this case is none other than Greece's cultural inheritance whose roots lay undisputedly in classical times. Moreover, the display of this inheritance through "choreographic, musical, and sartorial riches" (Shay, *Choreographic Politics* 239) orchestrated the cultivation of a national pride in owning this tradition. Other dances (or even songs in non-Greek dialects), whose character evoked cultures east or south of Greek national borders, were deplored in this ideological struggle to identify with European supremacy.

In closing, I revisit my title, "The Worlding of Greek Dance." Coined by Gayatri Spivak, the term "worlding" proves particularly useful in this reflective treatment of the process through which the Greek dancing body came to be defined (although "confined" is, perhaps, more appropriate). The term apprehends this process of definition and confinement fully. The example that Spivak provides to illustrate a moment of worlding is subtle, subtlety paradoxically enhancing its potency. A British soldier, named Birch, accompanied by a native escort, rides across the landscape of India in the early nineteenth century. He appears

> a slight romantic figure if encountered in the pages of a novel or on the screen. He is actually engaged in consolidating the Self of Europe by obliging the native to cathect the space of the Other on his home ground.... He is worlding *their own world*, which is far from mere uninscribed earth, anew, by obliging *them* to domesticate the alien as Master. Much "thicker" descriptions of this are, of course, to be found in settler colonies — a worlding visited upon "native" Americans, Black South Africans, Australian Aborigines, the Suomis of Northern Europe. (*A Critique of Postcolonial Reason* 211)

This passage tells of the multifarious ways in which the imperial project achieved its purposes. Spivak images the process whereby the "native" is instructed to assume the colonizer's notion of geographical, social, and cultural experience of his own "native" subjectivity.

My discussion in this chapter employs the dynamic of this image and extends the visitation of imperial worlding, in the terms that Spivak describes it, to Greek culture. Particularly in relation to music and dance, the emotional loading embedded in cathexis is a most appropriate evo-

"I have seen
this dance on
old Greek
vases":
Hellenism
and the
Worlding of
Greek Dance

cation since some forms of Greek music are revered, and quite rightly I believe, repositories of culture and history. Represented as colonized space, the Greek dancing body came into existence in an essentially Eurocentric world. The events which constituted its worlding were less subtle than the British soldier on an itinerary through the Indian landscape. These events were made up of, oddly enough, not the inscription on "a supposedly uninscribed territory" (*The Postcolonial Critic* 1) but the clearing of the palimpsest so that the classical script of antiquity would, supposedly, become discernible once more. This process of clearing and then rewriting the text that was to be uncovered, the glorious legacy of the ancient Greek past, were both components of the imperial project enacting itself in Greece. Indeed, as Spivak puts it, "this worlding actually is also a texting, textualising, a making into art, a making into an object to be understood" (*The Postcolonial Critic* 1). The palimpsest was cleared through a systematic (and systemic) application of state machinery that reprinted texts and spread the word of how the Greek body dressed; it celebrated a prescribed identity through kinesthetic motion. During its performance, the Greek body strives to negotiate movement between the poles of East and West as these were reified by Dora Stratou's discourse on the classical heritage and the advent of "Eastern" songs and dances—rebetika—from Christian, predominantly Greek-speaking populations from Turkey. The Greek dancing body was compelled to settle for a masculine, "European-identified" disposition, following an almost constant negotiating process involving the harsh legacy of Ottoman rule against the idealistic vision of Ancient Greece and the trauma of 1922. This is a process that I see as constant, a process of settlement that has to be reached continuously.

Imperial body discourse inscribed itself onto the Greek body in a manner that is contiguous with the treatment of the khawals, the ghawazee, the çengi, and the koçek. The Greek dancing body has been "worlded" with specific movement and confined expression. The dancing boys from the Greek islands, the same dancers that excited the Janissaries' erotic passions, have faded into oblivion. There is no trace of them while mention is rare. Homophobia manipulates the breadth of this invisibility and the rough texture of its silence. Nearhos Georgiades's treatment of the koçek provides a sad illustration. He describes the urban song and dance traditions in Epirus and the Thessaly plain of Northern Greece where male dancers seemed quite popular, and names some of the dances they must have performed and instruments they must have played. How-

157

*The Tsifteteli,
Grecian
Orientalism,
and the Male
Dancer*

ever, following the mid-nineteenth century, he finds that the Ottomans relaxed the restrictions on female performers so that the koçek began to be replaced with female performers. Georgiades feels that with the passing of the koçek, "things became *more natural*. The dancing boys were replaced by female dancers who played tambourines and zills and sang and danced in exactly the same manner [as the boys]" (my emphasis, my translation 30-31).

Angela Shand concludes her article by depicting a scene that blends Elias Petropoulos's verbal depiction of the female tsifteteli dancer and an actual phenomenon that is popular in Greek nightclubs:

> a woman dancing tsifte-teli on top of a table covered with glasses, plates and ouzo bottles, while below her admirers clap, shout encouragement, and throw flowers and paper money.... For many Greeks, the tsifteteli remains an Oriental dance of a woman without restraint: beautiful and sensual, but also dangerous and tempting. Placing the dancer on the pedestal of the taverna table may celebrate the sensual and exotic elements of her dance, but it also restricts her movements and allows others to keep an eye on her. Her potential danger is thus averted, and the tisfte-teli is made safe for Western civilization. (132)

That the tsifteteli has to be made safe for "Greek Westernness" has formed a significant part of my argument. Indeed, the dancer's physical constraint assuages Greek sensibility since such limitation contains her potency and even denigrates the artistic potential of this dance to merely exhibitionist spectacle as opposed to "empowering and subversive" ritual, as bell hooks describes it. However, the dancer is placed on the pedestal of the taverna table not only to recycle the traditional sexist notions, which are appeased by such shows of apotheosis of the female body, but also to divert the gaze of the spectators from each other and from the dance itself. With the dancer on the table, the dance is, in effect, erased. And the men fix their gaze on the swaying female body so they will not gaze at the sweaty foreheads and cleanly shaven cheeks of their male associates across the table, or imagine on their own bodies the possibilities and propositions engendered by every successive dance move.

6 / What Dancer from Which Dance?
Concluding Reflections

All of this bogus exoticism, this well-tooled suberoticism, would be in vain if it did not unveil what colonization cannot name, even if this unnamed seems to be satisfied with the extreme deformation that the postcard offers it.

Malek Alloula, *The Colonial Harem*

Rescuing the Exotic: Cults and Politics

May of 2001 saw the organization of a significant and ambitious event in the world of Oriental dance in North America: the Second International Conference on Middle Eastern Dance. Predictably, considering the magnitude of the event, the conference attracted hundreds of Oriental dance enthusiasts from all over North America as well as other parts of the globe, who crowded the campus of Orange Coast Community College in Costa Mesa California. There was a feeling of elation in the atmosphere, a sense of congeniality, of sisterhood (I was one of only a handful of male participants; hitherto affairs of "brotherhood" and heterosexual male camaraderie have held little charm for me). Compared with the conference style I have been accustomed to, this one featured an extraordinary line-up of engaging and exciting events. Apart from "academic" papers, there were film screenings, dance shows on two consecutive nights, presentations by Aisha Ali and Carolina Varga Dinicu (who have both devoted time to researching, performing, and documenting dances of North Africa), and dance workshops with the famous Egyptian dancers Nagwa Fouad and Farida Fahmy, and choreographers Mohammed Khalil

Notes to chapter 6 are on page 216.

160

*What Dancer
from Which
Dance?
Concluding
Reflections*

and Mahmoud Reda, all of whom are living legends in the world of this dance form.

The conference usefully addressed some of the harmful assumptions concerning the dance today in North America. Nevertheless, despite the celebratory atmosphere, tinged with a certain sincere and hard-earned glamour (considering the struggles of the dance), the problematic politics of the event and the treatment of the dance itself were discernible, if opaque. The crowd attending seemed to be predominantly white and decidedly middle class. There were, of course, the special non-white guest stars from Egypt, but even they breathed a certain bourgeois air, especially Farida Fahmy, who had completed an MA in Dance at the University of California at Los Angeles.

Directly pertaining to issues of race and colonialism were some disturbing and even disheartening moments that marked my experience of the event. Once again, I had to contend with an attitude that unfortunately enjoys an alarming amount of support in the community and which praises the belly dancers and instructors in North America and Western Europe as the sole carriers and perpetuators of the "authentic" Middle Eastern dance tradition. An overwhelmingly neo-colonial attitude permeates these assumptions. Paul Eugene Monty's commentary on the artistic consequences of Eastern participation in the World Exposition in Chicago in 1893 seems to intimate a sanctioning of this attitude:

> Proponents of the *danse du ventre* did not have the formalism, philosophy, or sophisticated backing for the promotion of their art. The dance, rapidly becoming associated with depravity, immorality, and indecency, seemed to completely disregard its possible pharaonic beginnings. If one could take the exoticism and uniqueness of this dance, and transform its artistic qualities into a form that was acceptable to the stage of the turn of the century, one could have a dance that would gather mass appeal. (89)

Marking the critical stages of the dance's introduction in North America, Monty further indicates the necessity of intervention in order to rescue those archaic elements that distinguish and validate this dance. Ultimately, he is suggesting a certain adaptation that will reform the dance and make it "acceptable," which, in my understanding, implies an apt commodification of the art for consumption in North America, this "stage of the turn of the century." In fact, he declares, "a group of terpsichoreans [sic] who became known as Salomé Dancers" with Loie Fuller as their predecessor, effected this transformation (Monty 89).

The conference was also permeated by a belief that circulates widely as knowledge, feeding this disconcerting neo-colonial attitude, that Egypt, the most significant, and geographically specific, reference for this dance, is losing its value as a resource location. The causes are, somewhat conveniently, traced to the Islamic "fundamentalists" (a term that in our contemporary context conjures the horror of Oriental fanaticism, anachronistic with Western modernity), who are becoming increasingly inexorable, ruining the dance scene and shutting down the clubs. An article that examines the dance crisis is Shareen el-Safy's "Raqs Sharqi: Cairo's Disappearing Act." In an informed and clear style, el-Safy offers the results of her on-site research on the complex reasons for the adverse developments in the contemporary scene of Oriental dance in Cairo:

> There are numerous reasons for these pervasive changes—some of the obvious are economics, religious conservatism and social fashion. Egyptians have less discretionary income because of high inflation and unemployment still plaguing them years after the Gulf War. The middle and lower classes are struggling to maintain their commitment to family and higher education while resisting Western mores. Their spending has become more conservative as have their religious leanings.... And there are some for whom neither money nor social standing is an issue, but going to a nightclub is simply *passé*—the trendy piano bars and exclusive, smaller clubs are more fashionable. (32-33)

In the article, el-Safy seems prepared, fortunately, to maintain an attitude devoid of those cultural assumptions and prejudices, and the hasty deductions that often flow from such perceptual weaknesses. That is, the causes that el-Safy identifies as contributing to the decline of Oriental dance in Cairo relate, obviously, to Western cultural imperialism as well as American military involvement and expansionist ambitions (the Gulf War and its adverse effects on the Egyptian economy are an obvious example of America's aggressive foreign policy that continues unabated, the invasion of Iraq being a recent example).

Despite interventions such as el-Safy's, many members of the North American dance community seem to thrive on the conviction that they are not mere guests to this art form. Instead, they assume the hegemonic role of emissaries who perpetuate, embellish, and safeguard its survival since, as they contend, Muslim fanatics marauding the land of the River Nile have no appreciation for their own artistic production.[1] Some people, perpetuating a clearly colonialist mentality, are not happy being guests to an art; they have to take it over and own it completely. Under such ide-

162

*What Dancer
from Which
Dance?
Concluding
Reflections*

ology the Orient is permitted to provide nothing more than an originary exotic inspiration, a promise of fabulous possibilities, but when it comes to the production of its own art forms, the Orient is denied any agency. Such ideological constructs want Oriental arts that enjoy some appeal in the West to be inchoate in form. If not inchoate in their native environment, then these arts have to lie in a condition of ruin or disrepair, abused by barbaric currents whose sway should be anticipated, supposedly, considering the tumultuous history of the region.

The grounds for such convictions are complex, yet they can be partly located in the strands of neo-colonialism. This has become a trendy and insidious way of picking up the banner of imperialism to continue the conquest, not in terms of administration or military annexation, but cultural imperialism. The problems that I complain about here on the subject of art have their parallel in women's issues. Voicing similar concerns but focusing on Islamic women's issues, Leila Ahmed asks, "how could the substitution of one culture for another be brought about for the peoples of an entire society or several societies?" She continues:

> In the debate about women in the Islamic world, as in other parts of the non-Western world, those proposing an improvement in the status of women from early on couched their advocacy in terms of the need to abandon the (implicitly) "innately" and "irreparable" misogynist practices of the native culture in favor of the customs and beliefs of another culture—the European." (129)

Similarly, the attempts of many followers of Oriental dance in the West have focused not simply on performing versions of this dance but in taking it under their guardianship, so to speak, as if to reimport it piecemeal to the places where it came from in the first place, considering its subsistence in the East as defunct.

In a rather peculiar turn of the dynamics of power, the travellers who ventured to inhabit and inscribe the Orient for the West have acquired, in contemporary Middle Eastern dancers' lore, an unforeseen currency in the economy of the Oriental "dream." Authors and other learned European men have become actors in the dramatization of the Orient's allure and mystic aura. Wendy Buonaventura is one of many devotees who have relied on such constructs (the alluring, mystifying "Orient," for example) to lend authority and stature to her performance work and her project *Serpent of the Nile*. Similarly, the back cover of Jalilah's compact disc *Journey of the Gipsy Dancer: Jalilah's Raks Sharki 3* features a text that seems intended to elicit a sense of yearning and nostalgia:

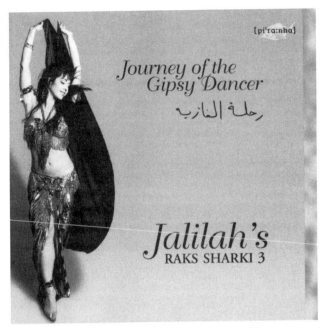

[pi'ra:nha]

*Journey of the
Gipsy Dancer*

رحلة الغازب

Jalilah's
RAKS SHARKI 3

CD cover, *Journey of the Gipsy Dancer: Jalilah's Raks Sharki 3*. (Courtesy Piranha Musik Produktion and Verlag AG, Berlin.)

Come and join the Journey of the Gipsy Dancer alongside the Nile; a journey which inspired such Orientalists as Nerval and Flaubert with the fascinating culture of the Ghawazee and their music. Listen to the authentic *Saidi* music soundscapes featuring some famous *Musicians of the Nile*. Let the remarkable music of *Raks Sharki* carry you into the world of the Egyptian Film, a world of sound that surrounded the fabulous singing and dancing moviestars [sic] like Oum Khalsoum, Samia Gamal and Naima Akif.

Jalilah, I should point out, belongs to a group of committed and consistent artists engaged in the live performance and recording of music for this dance. Also, her musical productions suggest meticulous and thorough study that is, fortunately, devoid of the offensiveness that has sadly become a common trademark of such productions.[2] Jalilah collaborates with some of the most experienced and respected Egyptian musicians. Her record company's dissemination of this art form, however, takes place within that same construct that has exoticized the Orient, seeking to filter its perception through the complicated lens of the European gaze. Advertising this particular production, *Journey of the Gipsy Dancer*, demonstrates a dependence on the problematic, and fortunately almost obsolete, term

164

*What Dancer
from Which
Dance?
Concluding
Reflections*

"gipsy," and its signifying layers of imperialist language production, thus mobilizing the familiar tropes that condense the Orient into one colourful and promising "authentic" package that refuses to heed temporal demarcations or historicity. *Journey of the Gipsy Dancer*, for example, is confident that it reifies a musical tour of the "Egypt of the Ghawazee," and "Flaubert and Nerval's Egypt." It also delivers the contemporary group "Musicians of the Nile" (which is a truly commendable ensemble of native musicians whose output is of great artistic value), and promises reminiscences of the golden years of the Egyptian film industry that featured the famous dancers named in the liner notes. To include Nerval and Flaubert in this context is a common and popular gesture in the pop culture that is born out of the love for Oriental dance in its contemporary renditions. More than any of the authors who have written about Middle Eastern dancers, these two literary personalities have been used extensively for their advertising potential, which has been exploited persistently because of its marketability. It invests the contemporary dance venture with an intellectual quality and a "seriousness"—legitimacy, in other words—thus quelling any anxieties concerning the art form's popular status.

Yet, in my mind, this discursive construction of a dance's reputation remains an interesting postcolonial sign because of what it implies and the notions on which it predicates itself. It relies on exoticizing these Western literary figures along with the Orient—a practice that suggests an ironic turn in Orientalist conventions. Moreover, Flaubert's involvement or experience with male dancers is rarely mentioned and only remotely alluded to. In fact, khawals or koçek do not often make it to album liner notes or explanatory booklets that accompany field-recording projects. This restructuring and remarketing of the dance as an overwhelmingly female art, and thereby preoccupation, has grafted itself onto the illusory image of the ghawazee. They become a useful and marketable feature, valuable because of its potential to generate exotica and perpetuate the romantic fascination for this tradition. As I point out in chapter 1, the terms for the dance are meant to invoke a certain lore that becomes the indispensable backdrop to the contemporary dance scene with researchers, enthusiasts, and dance instructors anchoring their pursuits in this imaginary.

Another interesting postcolonial sign is the adoption of "exotic" artistic pseudonyms by European and North American performers. Names such as Sheherezade, Zeynab, and Soraya, with the mystique they exude in the white mainstream, become a necessary (and expected) accou-

trement to the belly dance performance. Along with the jewellery, the costume, and the makeup, the exotic name bedecks the dancer who takes
to the stages of North America. On this issue of assuming a stage name,
Elizabeth Buck believes that "altering reality through masquerade can
be cathartic and is valuable in the maintenance of social and mental
health" (30). I find her allusion to Greek classical drama embedded in the
term "cathartic" important because it suggests seeing dance as a mimetic
ritual of sorts. Yet, often, this baptism (I am thinking here of the mystery
of baptism in the Greek Orthodox Church that is also a naming ritual)
that marks the passage into an artistic identity appears to contradict the
motivations of many of these enthusiasts' involvement in belly dance,
motivations which apparently originate from an (often vague) desire to
discover their body and its hidden sensual powers.[3] Iris J. Stewart echoes
this desire while describing a personal pilgrimage that allows her to journey "into the sacred feminine and the secret truths … about women's
spirituality," where she gains access to her female ancestors' "spiritual
wisdom" (1). I find Stewart's approach commendable (and I mean this in
earnest and not merely as rhetoric).[4] Nevertheless, I feel that it perpetuates certain problematic themes. I cite Deagon's sensible skepticism on
this theme, which she identifies as "revisionist narrative":

> The woman's expressive voice is still located in a place specifically Other:
> not only the orient, but the orient of the all-encompassing, distant past.
> Similarly, the new narrative highlights ideas of personal, yet universal,
> motions of self-discovery and self-expression, which perpetuate essential-
> ist ideas of woman as natural, timeless, and embodying. The definition of
> the dancer's place as individual, timeless and transformative distances
> her from areas of cultural interchange that vitally define her art in a
> broader cultural context. Perhaps most problematic are the gendering of
> Oriental dance as feminine and the wholesale projection of spiritual sig-
> nificance into its original culture; both readings may interfere with West-
> ern dancers' accurate appreciation of the dance in its primary milieu.
> ("Dance of the Seven Veils" 19)

I would like to concentrate on Deagon's problematizing of the Orient as
concept and posit certain objections regarding the charting of the East
in the contemporary dancer's journey.

For one, I find it alarming that, occasionally, the Mother Goddess cult
seems to entail oblivion to questions of empire, race, and class. A disci-
ple is fulfilled by the cult's conferral of "truths" and by the assumption of
another exotic name. This renaming enacts the "going native" motif.

Because this transformation takes place in an Occidental setting, the transgressive subject feels secure to embark on the quest for "spiritual wisdom" and also to indulge recklessly in this newly discovered "native" identity, flirting audaciously with primitivism and the concomitant peril that lurks in outlandish escapades enacted within the realm of the self.[5] In essence, this trajectory serves to affirm a colonialist principle and its perpetuating ideologies while preserving, as it runs its course, the hierarchical relation with the East in lofty statements such as "belly dance (by whatever name it is called) is poetry of the body expressed in ancient meaningful gestures" (Stewart 97).

What I am suggesting, in other words, is that the discovery of primeval truths in a dance tradition of the "Orient" (the scare quotes indicate the shift into modernity where the geographical Orient is not the Middle East anymore but a vague, floating concept) satisfies certain agendas that are connected to imperialism. The fact that these claims about Oriental arts are made under the rubric of feminism further complicates this particular type of domination. As Leila Ahmed argues,

> Whether in the hands of patriarchal men or feminists, the ideas of Western feminism essentially functioned to morally justify the attack on native societies and to support the notion of the comprehensive superiority of Europe. Evidently, then, whatever the disagreements of feminism with white male domination within Western societies, outside their borders feminism turned from being the critic of the system of white male dominance to being its docile servant. Anthropology, it has been said, served as a handmaid to colonialism. Perhaps it must also be said that feminism, or the ideas of feminism, served as its other handmaid. (154-55)

Indeed, colonialism championed a particular brand of conquering virility and male homosociality. Belly dancing transcends the conceptual divide of East and West so that its exponents are, in a sense, "outside their borders." Yet, in this location, the "new" dancers do not critique white male conquering masculinity or racial and sexual discrimination but are content, instead, to move with "ancient meaningful gestures."

Again, the ghawazee have been variously fashioned to provide a requisite backdrop to this experience. Apart from their commercial value and "exotic" inspiration, the ghawazee are made to assume choreographic poses as the threatening, sensual, othered women who have to retain their mystique as a foil to the character of this dance today. Crucial in settling this contemporary character is the taming of the dance's sensuality. The process of its taming for Western audiences and enthusiasts—these include largely white middle-class women able to afford time and money for classes—has been proud and insistent as well as rigorous.

There exists a parallel between the average performer of Oriental dance in North America and a tradition of Eastern embodiment by Western artists. The dynamics of this embodiment are particularly poignant on stage. Jane Desmond's analysis of Ruth St. Denis's *Radha* is quite relevant here. Desmond argues that St. Denis, as a white female performer dancing the East for a white audience, invites the possibility of psychological identification with the performer:

> Framed by the essentialist, transcendent spirituality of the piece, the audience is brought into ego identification with the white as nonwhite and the Western as Eastern. At the same time, the voyeuristic and fetishistic aspects of the dance (enhanced by its construction as spectacle) objectify it as separate from the observer. A "colored" white woman ... also evokes an ambiguous response. While "mixing" sexualizes the white woman, it simultaneously indicates a potential mixing of the race, legally proscribed at the time. If ideologies are based on binary constructions of difference necessary to the maintenance of hegemony, performance thus indicates the ambiguity of such binary constructions and their true dialectical function in the production of meaning. ("Dancing out the Difference" 48)

Of course, the process of assimilation that Desmond suggests for the audience vis-à-vis the dancer (ego identification with the Other while also experiencing it as being apart from their subjectivity) also happens within the dancer herself. Renamed and exotically adorned for her performance, the white North American dancer exposes the ambiguity of binary construction. Her assumed alterity embodies difference. Yet she also confirms the ideological binary by simulating interracial mixing and feeding with such images the "desiring machine" of colonialism.

In many cases, disciples acquire only the controlled and circumspect version of the art as disseminated by their dance instructors. With methods that seem to be informed by Dora Stratou's discourse on the threatening solo improvisational moment of the dancer, prevalent ideologies seeped into the perception and rendition of the dance, preventing it from being anything that is hitherto "uncharted," the term being significant as a metaphor for the space of subjectivity as well as Empire. I wish to rearticulate this disavowal in terms of desire and passion as Marta Savigliano explores them. Her theory formulates much of what I have tried to show in relation to Middle Eastern dance:

Desire is invested with legitimacy, the authority enjoyed by those in power;
Passion's power lies in its illegitimate nature precisely because it is imputed
to nature, to the primitive, to the irrational. Hence, Passion's power resides
in "empowerment," in seeking to partake (par-take) of some crumbs of
the power held in legitimate hands. Passion's power is akin to a terrorist
manoeuvre that asks for containment. It is wild, inhuman, beyond conquer-
able nature—that is, supernatural—and must be subjected to the workings
of the civilizing/humanizing Desire. Passion's doings are outside the realm
of History; they belong to the universe of Fate. Desire gives rise to subjectivity: desiring subjects who master Passion by making of Passion artifacts
and objects of Desire, which is permanently displaced, disembodied, and
reincorporated into someone/somewhere else—hence the Lacanian riddle
"desire of Other's desire, desire for the desiring Other." Desire follows and
replicates the avatars of conquest, civilization, and progress. Contrarily, Passion resides rightly by the dead end of survival. (10-11)

Desire is modern and charted. Passion is "anachronistic" and uncharted.
Kuchuk Hanem and Azizeh sing and dance and the passion of their
performance moulds the white subjectivity of Flaubert, du Camp, and
Curtis.

The out-of-control dancing subject that Dora Stratou tames in her
discourse is a passionate native who Stratou reinstates as a desiring male,
such as those who watch a woman dancing on the table at a Greek party.
"Forget Dora Stratou," Alkis Raftis exclaimed during one of our conver-
sations at a conference in Corfu in October 2002. "She's been dead for
thirty years!" he continued, urging me to move on in my exploration
unhampered by what (I assume from his comment) he regarded as defunct
discourses. She may indeed be dead for that long but her legacy is rooted
so deeply in Greek ideology that it will take several generations to unlearn
some of the autocratic teaching she has inflicted on us.[6] Her name
appeared on numerous posters at the conference and was highlighted
through several dance troops that operate under the auspices of the Dora
Stratou Dance Theatre. So ubiquitous was this name that every corner
of the Corfu Municipal Theatre seemed to reverberate with it and, by
extension, every corner of Greece. The refusal of many to acknowledge
the kinesthetic possibilities of the tsifteteli is a byproduct of her artistic
industry and yet another manifestation of the intricate ways in which
this particular dance becomes a performance of a complex matrix of
national, gender, sexual, and class issues.

Even the hybridity of the dance is not a popular subject of investigation when many dance instructors profess to teach the "pure and

authentic" Egyptian Baladi version of the dance. Not surprisingly, a large majority of the exponents of the dance today in North America are white, middle-class women who advocate for Oriental dance in the Iris Stewart mode. In a strong sense, Oriental dance in the West is predominantly a white endeavour and a white concern. Enthusiasts, who remain persistently oblivious to the wide-reaching effects of colonization, the history of oppression and exploitation of "Orientals," and the imperial domination of global affairs, become complicit with systems of oppression, which they perpetuate in the field of Oriental dance. This site of oblivion and lack of acknowledgement accommodates the privilege and support for neo-colonialism of these enthusiasts. Donna Carlton raises but does not pursue the same issue in a passing comment in *Looking for Little Egypt*: "the trivialization of Arab cultures continues today in the entertainment media's use of cartoonish ethnic stereotypes. This perpetuates cultural ignorance and provides ugly reminders of the colonial era" (19).

The conference performances closed with a percussive piece by Bassem Yazbek performed by "Jillina and the Sahlala Dancers," a group of remarkably slim and fit female dancers (slimness contrasts with dancers' images from the Middle Eastern past), all of them sporting luxurious coiffures and astounding talent. (I rely on memory for the details of the show.) The upbeat choreography was impressive because of its staggering precision, the finished moves, and the meticulous shimmies. Yet despite the superb choreographic composition that raised the roof, there was something slightly perturbing about this particular act. The next morning in the shuttle from the hotel to the conference site, Yasmina Ramzy—the accomplished dancer and teacher from Toronto and founder of the Arabesque Dance Company—helped clarify some of my doubts: "Oh, it's not Arabic," she affirmed, "but it's great," she concluded.[7] Indeed, by stating what the identity of the choreography was not, Ramzy helped me locate the roots of my larger concern for the recent trends in the interpretations of Oriental dance. I do not worry so much that they are not "Arabic"—whatever this might mean; I worry that the priority is on a white, middle-class performance of femininity, which is also decidedly heterosexual in its signification. Sexually unequivocal interpretations have become not only fashionable (this group had that particular look that accords an almost archetypal performance of what seems to be a traditionally male construct of feminine beauty: white, fit, dynamic and youthful) but almost required.

Jillina's closing act at the conference heralded a further development that was to take the Oriental dance world by storm. In 2002, Jillina became the artistic director of a rather controversial endeavour called "The Bellydance Superstars and the Desert Roses." Miles Copeland—the famous impresario who also managed successful pop bands like The Police and REM—engineered this project with the intention of tapping into a market that is, apparently, hungry for luxury, glamour, and exotica all blended into a spectacle. Belly dance provided a perfect theme for such an extravaganza. He recruited belly dancers who, in his words, "are not only brilliant at what they do, but they have a power on stage; they have a charisma; they have a smile that's infectious. They look good. Men and women want to watch them" (Gold C14). In order to pre-empt any possible complaints about aspects of the show, Copeland makes his requirements known: "I've said to everybody, 'I'm sorry. I need women who have a good look. And they have to have the stamina. And they have to be committed for nine weeks, which means they can't have a husband and three kids at home. This is the best-looking belly-dance troupe that's ever existed" (Gold C14). The emphasis on "looking good" and its definition is, of course, worrisome and it taunted Dondi Simone Dahlin, one of the belly dancers on tour with the troupe. In her diary, published on the Bellydance Superstars website, she records some of her concerns:

> Maybe he [Miles Copeland] is money hungry and doesn't really care about the girls as long as they are youthful and beautiful and making a good buck for him.... I have feared that he will perpetuate the myth that women have to be 22, thin and gorgeous to be successful... the exact opposite of what is so incredible about this dance form. Most of us have spent years in bliss that we found a dance where we don't have to have boob jobs and tummy tucks to perform and shine in public venues. We can be women and it has been honored in this dance.... I have also feared that I am the only one really talking about this ... that other dancers and teachers across the nation are still biting their tongues so they won't get on the bad side of Miles Copeland. There is a lot of butt kissing going on.

After voicing all these significant and very valid concerns, Dondi S. Dahlin assuages the readers of her diary that all was resolved following what *seems* to have been a heartfelt exchange with Copeland:

> Thankfully, many of my fears have subsided. I have had real visits with Miles and heart-to-heart talks about concerns and issues with this tour. Tears have streamed down my cheeks with exasperation in my voice. Through it all he encouraged me to speak and he listened. He has given

me quality time in voicing my opinions. Though he may never change his views about what a woman's beauty is and can be, I feel like I have been heard and that feeling can make the difference between me leaving the tour in anger and staying on with pride. (Dahlin np)

There does not seem to be a happy resolution to Dahlin's concerns here. From her words, I understand that nothing got resolved and the issues she confronted Copeland with remain largely unaddressed with the emphasis kept squarely on those dancers who qualify as "glamazons" (a new term, for me, with striking significations that seem to derive from show-business, mythology, and modern fashion stereotypes).

As could be anticipated, the Bellydance Superstars extravaganza occasioned a series of newspaper articles that describe the dance in tongue-in-cheek terms, such as Kerry Gold's article in the *Vancouver Sun* on 8 April 2004: "Impresario Miles Copeland is setting out to prove that the way to a man's heart is through the belly. A woman's taut, gyrating belly, that is" (C14). The potential for the dance to signify transgression or transformation, as in the cult of Salomé, still exists, of course, although now the priorities have shifted and some of that transgression and transformation vanishes before the sparkling veneer of such performance of fitness, unambiguous gender and sexuality, and precise choreography. Moreover, Copeland is confident and happy that his show appeals to different crowds. As Kerry Gold puts it in her article, "Bellydance Superstars appeals to the huge network of women who relate to the art form's empowering feminine qualities—as in those women in search of their inner goddess. Copeland's goddesses also happen to come with exquisite packaging. For the men in the audience, there's an abundance of cleavage and booty" (C14). The women in the audience, then, get to feed their imagination on the goddess potential, while the men get to feed their hungry gaze with an "abundance of cleavage and booty" so that everyone should leave this show feeling quite full. Of course, most disconcerting about this male ordering of things is that the women, again, are seen as unable to relate homosocially or homoerotically to another woman's dancing body (such relationship remains unspoken in the popular press), and have to remain fixated on some transcendental "goddess" ideal while the men, by virtue of gender and heterosexuality, are entitled to voyeuristic consumption of the performing female body—a consumption that will yield immediate pleasure and instant gratification.[8]

172

What Dancer
from Which
Dance?
Concluding
Reflections

Orientalist "Management" in Greece and Egypt

This glossy feminine archetype, as represented by the Bellydance Super-stars, has also become popular in Athens as well, where the best-known and most sought-after belly dancer, Eleonora, is a non-Greek woman (although, perhaps, not quite a "glamazon" since her legs may not be long enough to qualify and her waist may not be as slender). She is a talented and skilled dancer. Yet her popularity is instrumented not merely by artistic talent but by various imperatives, particularly the sublimated need to further distance this art form and its possibilities from the collective Greek imaginary. Both performances, her foreignness and her Oriental dance, have crucial implications for the embodiment of the dance in the Greek context.[9] Having or exhibiting no connection to rebetika, Eleonora removes this art even further for the average Greek by contributing to a certain foreignness. Therefore, Greek audience members will not need to focus on what their share in the legacy of this dance is and will not have to question their own participation in its artistic practice, thereby perpetuating a certain evasive and non-committal attitude towards this decidedly Eastern art form.

These modern appropriations are akin to efforts in Egypt to re-present an innocuous version of this dance. Mahmoud Reda, one of the celebrity guests at the conference and an Egyptian dancer and choreographer with enormous output, choreographed "hygiene," meaning desexualized, adaptations of Oriental dance. In his article "Parallel Traditions," Anthony Shay draws attention to the ways in which the Reda Folkloric Dance Company of Egypt, along with other international state folk ensembles, "attempts to mask the very overt sensuality for which Egyptian dance is famous" (39). In relation to male performers, Shay argues that this attitude stems from an embarrassment for cultural traditions. This embarrassment is directly related to the adoption of Western bourgeois attitudes (a pattern that I have examined closely in chapters 1 and 5 in relation to Greek dance). Reda's formalized interventions enact colonization from within, responding at the same time to the severe objections of the Egyptian elite:

> The elite and upper classes of Egypt typically expressed embarrassment toward their native dances in general and towards belly dancing in particular. One of the causes of this embarrassment is the impact the West has had on Egyptian culture. Many of the educated Egyptians to this day aspire to, and imitate the Western way of life. An example of this attitude ... is seen in Musharrafah's *Cultural Survey of Modern Egypt* in which

he wrote about dance saying that: "as school activity it is mainly Western: as 'swing' exhibitionism, it is an industrial product; as a Franco-Arab cabaret, it belongs to the tourist trade, and as a native vulgarity, it is a neurotic activity." (Fahmy 12)

Farida Fahmy played an important part in intervening and making certain shifts within this neat classification of Egyptian dance activities. Even though "the belly dancer was, to the chagrin of many Westernized Egyptians, the sole dance image that characterized Egyptian culture at home and abroad" (Franken 275), Fahmy, with her great talent and Western education, seemed to be the perfect artist to disinfect this sore image. As Marjorie Franken concludes, her moral irreproachability, modesty, and unprovocative performance rehabilitated and made respectable the image of the female dancer, thus offering fresh hope for the new national image of Egypt itself (279).

If Egypt needed a new and unprovocative national image, it was partly because of its colonized self-disavowal. Deriving his theoretical framework from Foucault, Timothy Mitchell suggests that Egypt was controlled not merely through an administrative imposition of discipline from above, but by successfully installing those mechanisms that generate discipline that flows from within the colonized body. More effective, therefore, than the exterior policing of individuals and their actions was the *production* of policed actions by the individuals themselves. Farida Fahmy's interventions in solo female performance in Egypt need to be examined in light of Mitchell's theoretical insights. That is, Fahmy and Dora Stratou have something in common: Stratou's projects achieved the purpose of re-presenting to the Greek people a package that contained not only their heritage, but also their ontology, what they should and should not be. This package was to be "unwrapped" from inside.

In a colonized nation, the most fertile ground for the cultivation of such discipline is the upper classes. Due to their privileged position, they would be the most responsive to British claims that the Empire moved into Egypt with the purpose of civilizing, educating, and refining this "savage" people. For a single, representative example of this discourse, I quote from Douglas Sladen's *Egypt and the English* (published in 1908). Among other assertions (he includes a chapter entitled "On the unfitness of the Egyptian to have representative institutions"!), he sees the indispensability of the English to this otherwise hopeless country: "In a word, Egypt needs the English because without them national bankruptcy would intervene with alarming suddenness, and Egyptian civilization would

174

*What Dancer
from Which
Dance?*
Concluding
Reflections

break down" (6). Elsewhere he expatiates on the noble British efforts to achieve some edification, often to conclude that such efforts are rendered futile by the limited intellectual means of the natives:

> To hear the Egyptian talk, you would imagine that his one desire was to improve his mind, to raise himself to the equal of highly-educated Europeans. As a matter of fact the Egyptian has no mind. Certain superficial notions and effects of civilization he assimilates—no coloured man imitates the collars of Englishmen so accurately; but in intellectual capacity and moral adaptability he is not a white man. (73)

The "perfect collars" that Sladen credits the Egyptian men with are a suitable enactment of what Homi Bhabha calls mimetic men—"almost the same but not white" (89)—although there do not seem to be any further signs that colonization will ultimately collapse in the face of this mimicry. According to Bhabha, "the *menace* of mimicry is its *double* vision which in disclosing the ambivalence of colonial discourse also disrupts its authority" (88). White supremacy has constructed itself upon the notion of the civil, the decorum of justness, the conduct of propriety, the educated intellect. Civilization resides within the overlapping space of whiteness, language, and strictly defined gender roles. Anything outside that space cannot aspire towards the same status. This is what Sladen is at pain to remind people when he declares "it must be remembered that an Egyptian is not a white man, but a mixture of black and yellow.... The Egyptian, whether he is a youth and wears comic-opera clothes and boots, or is one of the fat men who make cafés odious, is in his ideas of women, morality and truth, yellow inside at any rate" (116). The contempt that is clearly audible in Sladen's tone presents itself as a moral and social sentiment intended to motivate and subsequently confirm the colonial cosmic ordering. These emotions are, then, fundamental precepts in racist ideology and have functioned as such in colonial discourse.

Anthony Shay informs us that within a decade of the British takeover, Egyptians began to produce arguments against their own customs, a sign that matured fully in the treatment of Oriental dance. In 1903, Mohammed Hilmi Zayn al-Din published a book entitled *Madar al-Zar* (*The Harmfulness of the Zar*), criticizing the famous exorcistic ceremony, which is practised in a number of cultures in North Africa and the Middle East (Shay, *Choreographic Politics* 198). Significantly, the zar is performed mostly by women (although Magda Saleh cites instances of male performers), which would imply that its censure is largely directed at women's rituals as well.[10] In contemporary Egypt, Karin van Nieuwkerk finds that what troubles female performers most is not, as she puts it, an "Orientalist misrepresentation," but the denigration they suffer in the regard of their own society's middle and higher classes. In fact, with her project *A Trade Like Any Other*, Nieuwkerk aspires to ameliorate the performers' status and treatment: "by giving insight into their lives and backgrounds, I hope to generate more sympathy for female entertainers on the part of Egyptian as well as Western audiences" (1).

Governed by my own Orientalist notions about Greece and Egypt, I found the similarities that I have drawn between the two states surprising and unexpected. My discussion of the Eurovision Song Contest raised issues akin to how colonialist politics affected the treatment of the arts in Egypt. The ambiguous reception of Mariza Koch's entry and the objections raised against her participation and its presentation have demonstrated ways in which imperial discourse governs the creation of an artistic order that controls not so much the means of production as the means of representation, hence the embarrassment over the Greek entry felt by many Greeks and Cypriots. It is this kind of control that confirms European hegemony and brings about that anxious chasm that demarcates modernity from non-western anachronism. If it had taken place in the 1980s, Mariza Koch's intervention would have been termed "ethnic," the term denoting "a euphemism for such old fashioned terms as 'heathen,' 'pagan,' 'savage,' or the more recent term 'exotic,'" as Joann Kealiinohomoku so cogently puts it (546). In other words, past traditions, whose notions of the body are now considered antiquated, inhabit what Anne McClintock calls "anachronistic space," unless they are deemed to fulfill a certain marketable spiritual model. Modernity, with its properly revised performativity, saves us from embarrassment and discomfort by remaining firmly within the acceptable parameters of physique and movement—hence the approval that greets performances by women who, in the frame of the western model, appear dynamic, athletic, and youthful, epitomized by the large majority of the Bellydance Superstars.

In the midst of all that has survived and revived, the absence of dancing men is noticeable. What happened to all the Greek island boys, Dimitraki and Yanaki of Chios who performed in the taverns of Galata, inciting an amorous chaos, making the pasha's soldiers lovesick? They have been forced inside the airtight closet constructed by Greek cultural epistemology. They have been filtered out of oral narratives, their existence completely annihilated as if they never existed. They have been subject to Orientalism which, as Stathis Gourgouris points out, takes on the profound meaning of reifying "that which cannot submit to the logic of identity, and which, precisely because of its resistance, must be forced to submit by being construed as hopelessly condemned to eternal exclusion" (131-32). The dancing boys vanished in the hope that Greece would absolve itself of its Oriental past, yet the sacrifices have proven futile since the Oriental character of Greece survives and the tsifteteli is a prime site where this survival occurs. When Gourgouris highlights "coincidences" between European and "indigenous" Philhellenism and Orientalism, beyond their proximate signification within the same imaginary geography, he finds their intersection historically and theoretically revealing: "the love of Greece is the love of the West—as such, entirely incompatible with the Orient. For, precisely in dissociating itself from the Orient, Philhellenism reveals its ultimate discomfort with modern Greece, at least with modern Greece as a cultural reality" (Gourgouris 139).

This erasure of the modern cultural reality of Greece resonates with attitudes one encounters towards Egypt. I have already referred to Paul Eugene Monty's allusion to the possible pharaonic origins of the dance. Writing the preface to his daughter's study *Ancient Egyptian Dances*, Dr. František Lexa voices strong objections to modern interpretations of Egyptian dance:

> Some years ago I saw some modern dancing girls perform Egyptian dances. The common characteristics of all these dances were the insipid, jerky movements, anaesthetic postures, and abrupt turns of limbs. Although some of the girls asserted that it was the ancient Egyptian pictures of Egyptian dancers which they copied, I could not recollect seeing such movements and postures on any ancient Egyptian pictures. (Lexová 5)

That the "girls" themselves defended their art to Lexa in terms of an ancient tradition must be an instance of what Mary Louise Pratt terms "an autoethnographic gesture, transculturating elements of metropolitan discourses to create self-affirmations designed for reception in the metropolis" (143). Modern Egyptian dancers as subjugated subjects engage the metropolis's constructions of those it subjugates. They stand very little chance of success with Professor Lexa and his daughter Irena, who established that dance in ancient Egypt was purely a European affair. Lexová found that men in Pharaonic times "always danced with great spirit, bounding from the ground more in the manner of Europeans than of an Eastern people," and "some postures resembled those of our modern ballet, e.g., the pirouette was appreciated by the Egyptians thousands of years ago" (7-8).

However, Oriental dance in this project has exposed not merely the tenets of imperialist discourse on the one hand, and the art's transformative gift on the other; it has also revealed the means by which it may diversify its signs of excessive articulation. References to jewellery and makeup are ubiquitous and persistent in the narratives I have visited and I have argued for a way of perceiving them as complementing movement. In a slightly different but related fashion, finger cymbals project the dancing body into an aural dimension as well as visual. This artistry offers the dancer a form of transformation, as I indicate in my discussion of Nerval's "Dancing Girls." To focus on equivocations of performative attire in the context of coloniality and performance means to analyze the topic of makeup and objects of adornment in racial terms. For, apart from their artistic potential that can be examined in an aesthetic, Romantic context or explored for its creative implications, in a contemporary understanding of the issue, their intervention on the landscape of the body has had far-reaching implications for the colonizing West. More specifically, makeup, jewellery, and even embroidered material and costumes have become entangled in the discourse of empire and its ideologies. The fetishization of jewels (even of movement itself) as objects where passion converges feeds the spectator's desire while also manifesting his own contraries. Anne McClintock's treatment of the fetish, and her insistence on liberating it from what have become traditional psychoanalytic definitions in the second half of the twentieth century, opens up new possibilities for reading the fixations on the dancers' adornments:

> Far from being merely phallic substitutes, fetishes can be seen as the displacement onto an object (or person) of contradictions that the individual cannot resolve at a personal level. These contradictions may originate as social contradictions but are lived with profound intensity in the imagination and the flesh.... The fetish marks a crisis in social meaning as the embodiment of an impossible irresolution. The contradiction is displaced onto and embodied in the fetish object, which is thus destined to recur with compulsive repetition. Hence the apparent power of the fetish to enchant the fetishist. By displacing power onto the fetish, then manipulating the fetish, the individual gains symbolic control over what might otherwise be terrifying ambiguities. For this reason, the fetish can be called an impassioned object. (184)

According to this analysis, Kuchuk's necklace becomes the impassioned material object that becomes charged with Flaubert's longing. Observing it during the dance and then manipulating it during sex allows him some symbolic control of the experience: "Effect of her necklace between my teeth ... I felt like a tiger" (Steegmuller, *Flaubert in Egypt* 117). The excitement in viewing, touching, and feeling adornment in the Orient was augmented by its treatment in the metropolis. The construction of the visibly virtuous bourgeois woman presented a sharp contrast with the adorned and made-up Middle Eastern male and female dancers whose cosmetic interventions symbolized an opacity that was to be found only in the "curled and painted" prostitutes so frequently written about in the literature of the London poor by writers such as Henry Mayhew and William Acton (Grewal 27). Having satiated himself with an extended perambulation of colonized Algeria and an extended scopic inspection (and enjoyment) of native female bodies, Frank Edward Johnson turns to a Biblical passage to voice his rebuke and condemnation of Oriental ornamentation:

> The fate of the Ouled Nail, or dancing girl, of Biskra is often that described by the prophet Jeremiah: "though thou clothest thyself with crimson, though thou deckest thee [sic] with ornaments of gold, though thou rentest thy face with painting, in vain shalt thou make thyself fair; thy lovers will despise thee" (Jeremiah 3:30). (13)

These artifacts, while signifying liberation and ritualistic transformation in the context of kinesthesia, were exploited by the colonial gaze as a means to totally subjugate the racialized Oriental body; the body was controlled through the instruments of its own transformation.

Colonizing through the Viewfinder

In the words of Trinh Minh-ha, "translation, which is interpellated by ideology and can never be objective or neutral, should here be understood in the wider sense of the term—as a politics of constructing meaning" (127-28). Throughout this book, I have dealt extensively with the politics of constructing meaning in dance through the travel narrative and the treatise on folklore as ideologically inflected translations of the experience. The photograph, however, is more than a contested translation. The photograph is a medium where the will to dominate the dances of ornamentation and motion proved quite successful. Not long after its advent, the camera was used to incarcerate the dancer and the dance, signalling their ultimate subjugation. Because it thrives on the psychic, gestural, and spatial elements it moves through, dance is a text whose efficacy seriously diminishes if translated into a fixed single dimension. The viewfinder of the early Orientalist photographers sought to reduce the dancer and her art to one still frame, one meaning only, an attitude whose "savagery" is conquered with stillness and, subsequently, display. Emotions may dance even through stillness (suggesting that dance energy may certainly imbue a static pose as well), yet the immense legacy of photographs of awâlim and ghawazee present an often sad and debilitating inertia.[11] Depictions of male performers, or Middle Eastern boys in general, also exist. Joseph Boone cites the example of Wilhelm von Gloeden who capitalized "on the Orientalist motif of the beautiful Arab boy in his portrait series 'Ahmed 1890-1900,' which was reproduced as tourist postcards" (63). However, because of the taboo attached to homoeroticism, such postcards have not transited through European post offices as pornographic currency to the same extent. Photos of dancers from North Africa circulated in the West as an importation that depicts, quite literally, the conclusion of a battle that is already lost. The Oriental jewelled woman is deprived of her gaze and her dance, with jewels now signifying her subjugation instead of a metamorphosis.

Perhaps in response to the photographer's artistic composition, there is still a strange fascination that I experience as my eyes rest on the images of Middle Eastern dancers that have appeared alongside Frank Edward Johnson's article "Here and There in Northern Africa," and on postcards that circulated in Europe in the late nineteenth and twentieth centuries. I absorb sedulously every detail of the incarcerated body with a mixture of allure and sadness. My academic knowledge, my Cyprus experience, and my love for the dance and its performance rush against the emotions that my gaze generates as it settles on the body that undresses for its violation each time the images in the photograph expose themselves. The postcard's "bogus exoticism" (Alloula 92), however, works in tandem with the gaze that the postcard receives. Discussing these images, Rhonda Garelick uses the metaphor of windows (vitrines as she calls them) and suggests that "spectators gaze into these vitrines to find some kind of affirmation or reassurance that their own identities are unfettered, that their gaze can penetrate unilaterally" (115). Indeed, even the depicted subjects who are not staring at the lens (and, therefore, the viewer) — those who do not return the gaze and stay frozen instead, remain in their position of pornographic exploitation. In fact, the dancer who performs live and returns the gaze to the audience marks the potency of the Orient. The potential exists for the live performer to challenge kinesthetically the imperial subject, a dynamic that is impossible in the medium of

180

*What Dancer
from Which
Dance?
Concluding
Reflections*

the photograph. As Malek Alloula comments, in the static photographic pose "the dancers and musical performers do not appear in front of an audience. Rather, they perform the obligatory figures of a *ritual* whose hieratic nature suggests the idea of a place and a feast outside space and time" (89). The postcard, then, lifts the subjects out of their reality, forces them into an artificial environment, and endows their pose with some kind of sacredness that enhances, perversely, the hedonism of the composition. Through this exploitative visual scenario, the Orientalist postcard remains but an object of manipulation in the hands and eyes of the viewer.

There is an interesting moment during Colette's travels that exposes scopophilic politics and the returned gaze. The demands made of an Algerian dancer, Yamina, when she performs for Colette's entourage alter the dancer's scopic dynamics of the exchange:

> Like all the Ouled-Nail she danced using her arms and hands … flanks and the muscles of her energetic little belly. Then she stopped for a moment's rest, using the interval to undo the rose-bordered bodice, the wide-panelled skirt and the chemise of ordinary calico, for the guide insisted that she dance naked. Naked, she returned to the middle of the room between us and the two musicians, who had now turned their backs. The red of the fire and the sinister white of the acetylene flame disputed Yamina's youthful beauty, the slender beauty of a huntress, barely encumbered with breast or rump. She danced the same dances, knowing no others. But, because of her nudity, she no longer smiled but turned her gaze away from us and refused any longer to meet our eyes. She looked away and above our heads, full of a sovereign gravity and disdain, to seek the distant, invisible desert. (81)

The guide's request for Yamina to perform naked might be a moment of autoexotica—an attempt to give the tourists what they expect to see. It seems to me, however, that this same moment shares some similarity with the staging of a still, photographic pose. The Oriental subject has to be tamed somehow, either through nudity or stillness and exhibition, in order to diminish the efficacy of her gaze towards the imperial subject. In this scene from Colette, the "red of the fire" and the "sinister white" of the acetylene flame do more than contest Yamina's beauty. They speak of the violation itself in appropriate colours—sinister whiteness reddened by its desire.

Rey Chow has examined critical objections to the most famous collection of such colonialist postcards, Malek Alloula's *The Colonial Harem*. Chow deems Alloula's anti-imperialist charge as spurious and questions his absolution from a pornographic gaze upon the reprinted images of Algerian women. Chow argues that,

Because Alloula is intent on captivating the essence of the colonizer's discourse as a way to retaliate against his enemy, his own discourse coincides much more closely with the enemy's than with the women's. What emerges finally is not an identification between the critic and the gaze of the colonialist-photographer over the images of the women, which become bearers of multiple exploitations. Because Alloula's identification is with the colonialist-photographer, the women remain frozen in their poses. (131)

Chow's useful objections ought to challenge the way we view these photographs of dancers and colonialist attempts to reproduce them. Yet it is precisely her comment on the "frozen" pose that suggests the greatest disempowerment and disability of the Oriental dancer. Trapped and immobile, she loses what agency her bodily articulation might offer her. Chow, however, does not pay sufficient attention to Alloula's commentary on the postcards. In the section "Song and Dance: Almehs and Bayaderes," where the epigraph to this concluding chapter derives, Alloula posits sensitive protests to these depictions:

The almehs and bayaderes, captured in ridiculous poses without movement—shutter speeds were slow then—evoke only the dead figures of a ballet equally forlorn. They do not even have the grace of faded things. They spin around, puppets of a tedious and repetitive imagination that is blocked in the dismal reiteration of its obsessive leitmotif. In so doing they reveal the fragments of a truth that, for the time being, attaches itself to their opulent and impudent bosoms, depicted in a manner calculated to delight a bad taste that is as brutal as it is pedestrian. (92-93)

Nevertheless, and since this project is very much about seeing and ways of seeing, Chow's comments have sensitized me to think about whether I too have taken advantage of the dancers, especially Kuchuk and Azizeh. In my research on Kuchuk Hanem, it took time to admit to myself that what drove me was a desire to search for her in the libraries and in the remnants of performed dance moves, just as Curtis and Flaubert searched for her in Upper Egypt. Throughout my quest, I felt tempted to surrender to an irresistible urge to romanticize her. I felt frustrated that descriptions of her vary greatly, as if writers are describing a different person entirely, because I needed to retrieve her, recuperate her, reinstate her as a carrier of culture, and valorize her dance technique—as if Kuchuk needs any of this. Most challenging—and disconcerting—of all was the realization that I have also been motivated by a longing similar to Flaubert's: to embody her. As I read the details that sketchily reconstruct

182

*What Dancer
from Which
Dance?
Concluding
Reflections*

her house in Wadi Halfa, in Upper Egypt, I resorted to my experience of traditional Cypriot architecture in an effort to draw upon the physical similarities between the two places as if such "likeness" could produce an intimation of Kuchuk or some of the atmosphere in which she lived and danced. Memory and imagination gently probed the details, hoping to yield some image of her house and a vision of the shadows of her courtyard as the afternoon sun lowers in the sky above the Nile. My quest for Kuchuk may have yielded her choreographies, but only in the signs they have left on the male bodies that have watched them, imperial signs and imperial retellings of the dance.

Have I simply displayed the dancers once again for public view, reproducing in quotations and epigraphs the same narratives that have trumpeted their scrutiny and exploitation? I embarked on this project motivated by the personal questions I explore in my introduction and a concomitant desire to intervene in the way the gaze behaves towards the body performing Middle Eastern dance. I am conscious of the fact that my own gaze is not innocent or pure. Like the viewer of pornographic postcards, I am confronted by my own projections. The postcards are pornographic because of what the photographer and viewer project onto them. "Intercourse" with these depictions involves precisely what the term implies: a communicative exchange between the viewer and the image. In other words, the viewer also shares a large part of the responsibility of how s/he will look at the photograph. These images involve a process of signification that goes beyond the reading clues of the colonizer and the pornographer/photographer. Nasrin Rahimieh's comments are helpful in this regard. In Alloula's account, Rahimieh sees an ironic turn whereby the photographer himself becomes the victim of his own unrealizable fantasies. Similarly, the viewer who expects sexual gratification from the postcards is not much more than an obsessively neurotic voyeur (40).[12]

My work tries to emulate Alloula's postcolonial readings of the postcards. Our projects rely on a will to produce the absent gaze, to rewrite the absent text of the photograph and of the dance. In the words of Ali Behdad,

> such work is an exercise in remembering, a recourse to a repressed memory that history has swept away, an anamnesia that produces new histories of resistance through speaking about the lack of a returned gaze in the history it tells. Alloula describes his text as a personal "exorcism" that thwarts the desolate gaze of the colonizer.... Such an anamnesiac prac-

tice is the opposite of the nostalgic histories of colonialism that have been and are in vogue today. (8)

I complain about certain contemporary attitudes towards Oriental dance because they qualify as "nostalgic histories." By contrast, my insistence and effort to "read" the choreographies of Kuchuk, Azizeh, and Hassan qualify, I hope, as "anamnesiac practice."

Focusing on dance is like focusing on an already vanquished text. Its loss, however, must not incite mourning. Dance is a text that inscribes itself on the body and in the air. We need to lose it in order to retrieve it. Perhaps there may have been a time when our imagination processed dance differently—again, I do not mean to lament this loss but to attempt alternative ways of seeing and thinking about seeing. Ultimately, we want to make dance's significations into a text that can be readable and memorable. Every performance I endeavour generates questions, doubts, and critique. Does my performance contribute to an exoticization of my body, or an exoticization of the music? Isn't what I perform a dance that I learned formally in North America? When I perform, does my audience have a context for the music and the choreography or do I violate both every time? Also, how do those diasporic members who originate from that enormous geographical expanse, the Orient of imperialism, relate to my show? Ali Behdad makes the following important assertion: "That Orientalism as a Western discourse on the Other continues to operate so powerfully only makes the need for counterrepresentational practices more urgent" (viii). If Middle Eastern dance in the West is often another way to propagate Orientalism, then how confident can I be in my earlier assertion that my dancing qualifies as counterrepresentational practice?

Beginning dance classes was a moment when I finally dared take action and invest my desire with a material form as I began to articulate my passion in spatial steps and bodily movement. The experience makes me comprehend that what guides and simultaneously drives my bodily articulations is the consciousness of a necessary utterance that implicates my gender, my sexuality, and my ethnicity. The constant shifts of my frame through the dance corporealize my resistance. My jewelled wrists and my coined hip scarf assist me by providing that space I need for my attempt; so do my finger cymbals as they slice rhythmically the air around me with sharp surges of rhythm. Performing is an attempt to superimpose a contrapuntal reading of my body's construction.

This lengthy journey into an embodied art form has also disclosed how signs of Orientalism and sexuality underlie my postcolonial experience.

The stereotype of the "lustful Turk" (which throughout my life, especially during my army service, I secretly found quite appealing and fascinating) and homosexuality were both invested with analogous horrors and revulsions. The tsifteteli manifests such "horrors" for me but transforms them, allowing me to surrender to what amounts to a kinesthetic deliverance from social proscriptions. In Cyprus, sexuality and nation are complicated and interwoven. British rule is the period when the extreme animosity between the two communities and the flagrant racism of each side grew tremendously. Apart from the seeds of racism, British rule has also sown the seeds of a contemporary masculine sexual crisis. Both during and following the years of the British occupation, hangings, killings, and beatings of young men involved in the national struggle (many of them hardly eighteen) were valorized and narrated endlessly as epics of remarkable adroitness and heroic national sacrifice. "Dying for one's country," Anderson says, "which usually one does not choose, assumes a moral grandeur … it is felt to be something fundamentally pure" (144). Indeed, pure and true patriotism cannot be contaminated with perverse passion and deviant erotic longing. Furtive encounters between Cypriot men and British soldiers in Kyrenia, or sex in the hammams (Turkish-style bathhouses) of Limassol or the parks of Nicosia, are condemned to a perpetual silence. The Cypriot body can be remembered and paid homage to only when in a state of punishment and reduced corporeality, but never in a state of hedonistic, homoerotic absorption. The history of these corporealities has been condemned to the same obscurity that has shrouded the Greek dancing boys of Constantinople.

Similarly, individuals with dissenting sexualities, such as myself, sought to realize their proscribed desires in Western metropolitan centres. These centres have been singularized into an accepting and permissive site of sexual exploration, often in fact, idealized as locations that foster alterity. Indeed, such perceptions represent an ironic reversal from the Orientalist ventures of European men seeking the polymorphous sexuality of the Orient. Since the proclamation of the republic, the Cypriots who emigrate are not only those in need of employment or a more prosperous future. Men and women of dissident sexuality seek to escape the confines of the island's closet by relocating to mainly Western metropolitan centres. Here, they imagine a community where they can desire and pursue fulfillment away from the tight restrictions of family and tradition and explore the privileges of citizenship in a queer nation. Such escape may yield a sanctuary but could also be nothing more than compelling exile with that "touch of solitude and spirituality" as Edward Said so sensitively puts it ("Reflections on Exile" 181). Whatever the case, exile or liberation, sanctuary or deprivation, such migrations beg to be studied and theorized further. Having assimilated Orientalist discourse and sexuality in these ways, I find the most use in postcolonial theory that combines postcoloniality and sexuality. Volumes such as John C. Hawley's *Postcolonial, Queer* and May Joseph's and Jennifer Natalya Fink's *Performing Hybridity*, closely examine gender and sexuality in a postcolonial condition, and thus enrich and advance Said's *Orientalism*, which, although radical and enormously influential, remains securely anchored in a masculinist frame of reference.

In the travel literature I have examined, "science and sentiment code the imperial frontier in the two eternally clashing and complementary languages of bourgeois subjectivity" (Pratt 39), and Oriental dance moves enact a fundamental motif in this clash. It was a stirring moment when I listened for the first time to the tsifteteli from Mariza Koch's album "The Coast" (Τα Παράλια), a title referring to the Ionian coast and its Greek populations. The late Stefanos Vartanis, a virtuoso from Asia Minor, played violin on the album. Moving to it makes me conscious of how I need to embody both theory and performance if I am to reclaim what I have lost in the history of colonialism and neo-colonialism. In her closing remarks to *Performing Hybridity*, Fink concludes the collection of essays in language that aptly describes my own endeavour:

> The pasts remembered here are deeply personal and idiosyncratic. Yet, they also speak to the yearning for affiliation with a collective history beyond individual formations. These are highly politicized stories, infused with questions of cultural citizenship, national and postcolonial identity, bloodshed, longing, and genocide that have been allowed only to ghost the borders and margins of the grand récit of official histories. (248)

Apart from being very appropriate, Fink's comments remind me of "Book 11" of *The Odyssey*. Odysseus, consumed by *nostos* (his longing to return home), travels to the Underworld to sacrifice to the ghosts of the deceased and hear Tiresius's prophecy. Following his libations and sacrifices, the ghosts emerge from the darkness of Erebus to drink from the stream of blood—a powerful scene that I envision as a stirring choreodrama. In a sense, this project has also been a choreodrama of sorts, an attempt to offer sacrifice to the ghosts whose utterance I need to invoke. As my hips negotiate physical space for those complex kinesthetic utterances necessary in this dance, what my body enunciates is the weaving and unweaving of these narratives—or, rather, the coiling and uncoiling of the colonial and postcolonial serpents, which writhe not because I seek to deliver my body from their control, but because they need to induce in my body an oracular utterance that will prophesy their joint fate. It is a ritual performance for the ghosts that roam the fields of Cyprus: Greek, Turkish, Greek Cypriot, Turkish Cypriot—shadows whose sighs imbue the earth, the stones, the moon itself, with grief and longing. When will these ghosts drink their fill of kinesthesia, and speak the dance?

And when they speak, what language will that be in? I come from an island that is divided between north and south. The zone of separation, the Green Line, is an eerie no-man's land with wild vegetation and derelict buildings that still bear the bullet holes from the fighting of 1974. In people's gardens, sacks of sand used in the battles are still piled up, the material wearing out and the sand pouring out. The north has remained "Oriental." Tourists describe it as a time capsule, a place where everything has remained frozen in place, unchanged: the sandstone buildings, the palm trees, the corroded gates, and rotting door frames. And just across the Green Line, the rest of Nicosia sprawls beyond the Venetian walls. It sprawls with its technology, its offshore company offices, its traffic jams, the picturesque reconstruction of its old quarter, mainly shops and restaurants for tourist consumption. I have talked about Middle Eastern dance and the performance of "sex," race, and nation. I have performed this entire project mostly in English, a language I strove to acquire as a means of escape from the confines of my construction. "Discussions of linguistic performativity," Eve Sedgwick tells us, "have become a place to reflect on ways in which language really can be said to produce effect: effects of identity, enforcement, seduction, challenge" (*Tendencies* 11). In this project, however, not only English but dance also has afforded a performance of my "sex," my race, and my nation. The semantic force of terms has determined my position but dance moves have shaped its sense. Mousbah Baalbaki, the male Lebanese belly dancer (along with other dancers who also struggle with audience and art and who remain unnamed, unacknowledged, and often unlooked at), also performs his masculinity, race, and nation in the midst of devastation, near Jerusalem, a divided city like Nicosia. In the face of the devastation and the irreparable damages to the postcolonial land, the transgressive and excessive moves of Oriental dance must remain untameable.

Epilogue

D*ancing Fear and Desire* has balanced itself delicately on the ambiguity that the phrase engenders. Through the pages of this book, fear and desire have danced with each other and solo, spinning through the sites that define and redefine them constantly, seeking absolution and also consummation. Simultaneously, the body that has performed this project has danced its fear and desire with every move feeding on the overlapping and ever-shifting territory of their dominion. I have endeavoured to demonstrate the intricate manner in which kinesthetic motion has formed the site of unique possibilities and transformations in the imperial realm while it has also signalled difference and pronounced forbidden yearnings. I have indulged autobiographical impulses while addressing issues of representation, national and sexual identity, and politics of movement in the performance of these identities.

In exploring conforming and errant kinesthetic narratives of Middle Eastern dance and colonialism, this book aims to contribute to three related areas of critical debate: queer studies, postcolonial theory, and dance studies. In the words of theorist and performance artist David Bateman, "queer theory reveals the vulnerability of the speaker, the subjects, and the issues he or she responds to, and all of the gaps and fissures that exist within popular consciousness regarding gender, race, sexuality, and the body."[1] My attempt here has been to delve into and explore these spaces. We have seen how mainstream Western scholarship has employed various standard responses to body-centred endeavours and experiences. If it could not deny or repress them, it would exoticize them. There is a lucid parallel here with the treatment that racial minorities, colonized peoples, lesbians, gays, and other marginalized groups continue to receive. To develop a theory of body-centred activities means, for one thing, to

Notes to epilogue are on page 218.

attempt a fresh approach to postcolonial inquiry—an approach where the questions are posed not by an unmoved subject but by a body that resonates with the object of study and embodies the misapprehensions and neglects of the past. The body and its movement demand a scholarship that, in the words of Susan Foster, "detects and records movements of the writer as well as the written about, and it places at the center of investigation the changing positions of these two groups of bodies and the co-motion that orchestrates as it differentiates their identities" ("Choreographing History" 16). This form of scholarship, that Foster appropriately names "ambulant," has already been undertaken, quite successfully, by critics such as Gayatri Spivak, Marta Savigliano, bell hooks, Trinh Minh-ha, and Susan Foster. They have challenged a significant part of the "epistemic foundations of canonical scholarship" (Foster, "Choreographing History" 12) contesting dichotomies such as theory versus practice, thought versus action, or logos versus body. I will be satisfied if this book makes even a minor contribution to ambulant scholarship.

Without this analysis of what Jane Desmond calls "a kinesthetics of sexuality" ("Introduction" 7), how is one to discuss contemporary incidents of human sacrifice? And I mean sacrifice here in its raw, brutal reification. A Queer Planet e-mail alerted us to a news item from Nigeria, titled "A Gay Murder in Jigawa," describing yet another homophobic hate crime. This crime becomes a tragic reminder of this project's purpose. The dubious journalistic manner in which the crime is retold through effeminaphobic narrative quickly becomes a specific example of the same kind of phobia that restricts the male "dancer" in his daily performed physical task. I focus on those parts of the tragic story that relate the bodily inscriptions of the unfortunate twenty-one-year old Innua Yakubu: "When he walked from his Mang hostel to the classroom, he picked his steps gingerly and wriggled his waist as a teenage girl. At night, after prep Yakubu would make up like a lady ready to meet his 'lover' at a secret rendezvous in Tsoho Gari not far from their hostel." The meanings his body wove signalled his sacrificial call. He embarked upon that dangerous kinesthetic moment when our quest for physical and spiritual fulfillment (a quest often fraught with fear, hesitation, and, quite often, the anxiety of imminent disappointment) becomes a threat to others who return the threat upon us: "Unknown to Yakubu, many of his friends, enraged by his effeminate attitude in school, planned to turn his fun into a tragedy. A group of sixteen boys followed him as he ran to meet his lover ... beat him with sticks and koboko until he could not move again."[2] But Yakubu's spirit, as part of a tragic, homophobic legacy that I dare say postcolonialism has universalized, will continue to inform the loss that I speak of in my work. He is a ghost of the past, yet as a body that has choreographed a certain history, he can put into motion the bodies of all those who would observe his written body.[3]

Belly dance, as I understand it and perform it, seems to be a survivor of constant struggles, which it represents and which also generate a certain sadness that forms a significant part of the general process of "authoring" dance. Freud suggests that the pathologized notion of melancholy implies the loss of a physical and/or emotional "object" of desire with melancholic dispositions infusing even the potential for present joy. Revisiting Freud's theory, it becomes evident that it applies to my moment of nostalgia for a reconsideration of the originary bodily theft—robbing my body of what have been traditionally considered "feminine" gestures. Recuperating loss is a kind of productive melancholy because within the kinesthetic moment the anamnesis, for me, is still—always already—present, thereby formulating a kind of emotional postmodernism that insists upon the presence of the past—the bodily presence—within each corporeal stance. I will persist in my attempts to retrieve the stolen joy of a liberated body from an oppressive, at times murderous past—the turning of a system of past/present oppression into a liberating present/presence: bodily presence, as in the dance.

For many of us, Oriental dance has played a soteriological role in our lives. Many are those who are aware of such potential in this dance—as if by some instinctual drive it seems at times—and anticipate its takeover. They search the gaps, the silences, those invisible spaces for traces of what they are forbidden to perform and feel. It is precisely within these interdicted, taboo sites that they will find the only place that can accommodate them, the place that will liberate those currents of passion and send them circulating throughout their being, depositing sediments of vital meaning in the remotest regions of their transnational and "transethnic" psyches.

Initially, I had not imagined that I would write this book and include any of my personal experience in it. Now I am surprised by how long and how overtly I appear onstage and I feel frustrated by how brief, shy, and even awkward these appearances are. My presence seems dictated by a strange ambivalence over which my consciousness seems to have had little control. On its own accord it sought to participate and on its own accord it sought to hide. What is the purpose of such oscillation? I am used to hiding and being unobtrusive as if my story will hurt less if it remains unheard. Traumas? No, not me; others have them. I don't suffer from traumas that need to be silenced. This work is about my own erasure that I attempt to reclaim through a dance that is also erased in many ways. More than I ever anticipated, my exploration of the topic soon had me weaving my steps and hips toward the sites of everything that hurts. Dance is capable of forcing such confrontations, which are hurtful as much as they are joyful and didactic.

Geographies of Dance

I will close with a series of brief acts that cite moments of geographical positioning and evoke rites of transformation and remembering, crossing and transcending. Ultimately, I want these moments to speak of the numinous dimension of kinesthetic experience. These acts are not meant to be read as vignettes to conclude this book. On the contrary: they are meant to dance the conclusion into new openings and choreographies that unfold below and beyond—not an exit but an en-trance.

Χόρεψε μου Τσιφτετέλι ("Chorepse mou Tsifteteli") 12 July 2001

It is early afternoon and I am spending some time in a rather dark stall in the men's room at the Lakeside Rydges Hotel in Canberra, Australia. No, I am not here to use the bathroom, but to thrash out my predicament over my course of action. This is the thirteenth ACLALS (Association for Commonwealth Literature and Language Studies) conference and its broad theme is resistance and reconciliation, a theme that appropriately sums up my own process. I am here to present a paper on belly dance and Cypriot masculinity. The complication is that I want to perform a tsifteteli as part of my presentation but the difficulties and impracticalities of such an endeavour weigh me down, making me resist—strongly—the possibility, while also wanting it badly. Some voice from a remote region of my mind repeatedly harasses me with "people do not go to conferences to belly dance but to present formal academic research so what do you think you are going to accomplish by such a foolish intervention in the tradition?" I don't answer. Grumpily, I pull up my harem pants, tie my coin belt around my hips, secure it with safety pins, and cover up my attire with a pair of broad formal pants that I wear on top. Pushing the stall door open, I make my way to the presentation room with my coin belt rattling in competition with my trepidation, both audible and both wanting (transitively and intransitively).

In my paper, delivered before a full audience, I delineate belly dance as an enabling site that helps me reconcile what my identity as a Greek-Cypriot man interdicts. The portable stereo I carry is queued to Roza Eskenazy's Χόρεψε μου Τσιφτετέλι ("Dance the Tsifteteli for Me"), a song with lyrics that are a fairly simple and common expression of love and an invitation for the beloved to arrive soon.[4] Nonetheless, this song also reflects the history of Roza's hybrid cultural embodiment since it includes verses in both Greek and Turkish. Despite doubts and insecurities about the endeavour (all that harassment from within), I proceed, confident that my audacious attempt is necessary if I am to project my body as text to be read (by me and by the audience) and in the process, I contravene the normalized conference attitudes. I press "play" and, rendered in the poor sound quality of a portable tape recorder, the bouzouki and Roza's voice fill the air, unapologetic and unselfconscious about their incongruity. Before a perplexed but sympathetic and kind audience, I drop my formal pants and free my hips to pronounce memories from childhood, remembrances of Roza's aged face on black-and-white TV, but also of her belly dancing (especially her fabulous pelvic drops) that was vigorous and pained, mature yet youthful in its character. I follow up with a self-critique of my performance and my Orientalist attire. However, I do not own up to how gratifying and liberating it has been to employ the seduction of the song in order to mark an alternate trajectory, in that room in Canberra, with sumptuous undulations and extravagant motion.

Corfu, Greece, November 2002

Between 30 October and 3 November 2002, Corfu hosted the Sixteenth International Congress on Dance Research organized by the Conseil International de la Dance (CID). Although fortunate to have had my proposal accepted and my paper published in the proceedings, I cannot forget that I conducted my correspondence with the organizers with some trepidation since I was uncertain about the reception of my paper proposal on the tsifteteli. Many times I have witnessed Greece's staunch intransigence in the politics of culture. Although the country is a land of contradictions and of a wonderful and very productive chaos in matters of culture, identity, and belonging, the mainstream ideology of Greece holds tightly the reins of conservatism and may, at times, prove a formidable opponent to artists or intellectuals who seek expression through alterity or who attempt to chant verses other than the well-rehearsed, approved refrain. This conference was going to be my first experience presenting my work on Oriental dance and my legacy of it as a Greek Cypriot in a Greek environment. My proposition to bring the tsifteteli to the forefront as a unique and valuable site of individual expression, not only of ethnic but also of gender identity, promised to make my presentation a test and a challenge. I had to prepare for battle at both fronts: the national legacy of the tsifteteli and my right to it as a man desiring to perform it. I did not even want to consider the queerness issue—that was a subject too formidable to broach.

When the moment came for my delivery, my disenchantment with what I felt was a general feeling of complacency and conservatism at the conference incited me to assail my unsuspecting audience with a brief choreography (not accepted in this conference canon as a conventional component of "academic presentations") and the following provocative statements:

I like dance that is erotic, taboo, proscribed.

I am not interested in what they present me with and tell me "this is your tradition, your heritage, your culture." Instead, I search the gaps, the silences, those invisible spaces for traces of what I am forbidden to perform.

I find the idea of Classical Greece sexy but not very useful.

I detest the sexism that ruins perfectly the things I love.

Authenticity is not my priority. I like hybridity, experimentation, infidelity, transgression.

The responses to my audacity were quite interesting and conflicting; at once uplifting and encouraging but also disheartening (what did I expect, really? I went looking for it!) Indeed, there was a small number of totalitarian men whose objections sought to dominate the atmosphere of the question period (I purposely kept my paper brief and invited audience comments and questions). They claimed not to be convinced and despite all my arguments insisted—without really arguing their position—that "it [the tsifteteli] still looks better on a woman." Of course, such an attitude is not simply obstinacy. It insinuates sexism as well as homophobia. The female body, denigrated by male control and social definitions, is easier to control than the male. And, of course, the last thing heterosexist men want to observe is a male body indulging in the pleasure of swaying and undulating movement. One of the Greek men, a folk dancer from Peloponnesus, posed a question by introducing it in such a way that made my ideas and positions seem "picturesque" and "eccentric," as if that outlook was a purpose in itself. This was, of course, meant to disarm me by diminishing the efficacy of my argument. Finally, the session chair, a math professor involved in Greek folk dance, objected (in fact, he looked offended) to my calling Ulf Buchheld sexist and ran to defend this German scholar whose research sought to confirm the ancient Greek roots of the tsifteteli.

A number of audience members were keen to point out that what I performed in my brief choreography was "Oriental," not tsifteteli—asserting the notion that there is a set and distinct vocabulary for the tsifteteli. Although there are certainly differences in the interpretations of the two related dance forms, such objections seem to signal a wish to say what the tsifteteli *is not* but not what it *is*. Greece, Cyprus, and the belly dance communities in the West present great variations in its performance, but what troubles me is the reluctance in my own culture to attempt interpretations that the music can certainly accommodate (if not incite) although the performers do not articulate. (I lament the absence of the shimmy in particular.) Perhaps this might be one reason why people often distinguish between "Oriental" and tsifteteli although, it seems to me, that in claiming ownership of a particular "brand," Greeks are guarding national and cultural spaces. In fact, the difficulty in defining what *it is* brings the indeterminacy of these spaces into sharp relief.

Despite these critiques, "Oriental" or not, there was an overwhelming response from a large number of people whose allegiance was firm and delineated a clear and strong sense of not only an international but also Greek-identified community of lovers of this dance. Responsive and supportive were many Greek women who made a point of approaching me to relate their fascination with my topic, to express excitement over my presentation, and to confess a secret but strong desire to learn complex renditions of Greek tsifteteli music (I suppose these complex renditions would qualify for what some of my audience termed "Oriental" and not tsifteteli). These confessions poured forth with such sincerity and eagerness that I was moved to see how profoundly this particular idiom of dance movement touched certain people. Are these people also searching the gaps, the silences, those invisible spaces for traces of what they are forbidden to perform and feel? It seems that these interdicted, taboo sites, as I have called them, hold out some promise of artistic expression and emotive accommodation.

Dawn in Belgrade, 6 July 2003

I am lying in bed in this somewhat shabby room of a hotel located in an old neighbourhood of Belgrade. From the large window behind my bed, I watch the first light of dawn stir on the horizon and spread over the buildings, over their grey walls, aluminum windows, and dense antennas that crowd the roofs. My body has remained wide awake through the whole night, pulsating, remembering, longing with Oriental dance. Every performance, however short or insignificant in the general scheme of things, sends every atom of my body into a mad, relentless orbit as if the speed and the intensity will trace, isolate, and eliminate each aching cell at once. I danced tonight for the first time, not to recorded music but to the rhythmic clapping of my audience and to the rhythms of my finger cymbals.

One member of my audience was a very young and compelling Slovenian man. His posture had something of refined grace, his beauty smooth yet robust, boldly marked yet unresolved as if sculpted by an awed but skilled and adoring hand. What drew me most strongly were his arms—long, graceful, murmurous—with an abundance that moved me, and curves stunningly, gorgeously defined. His skin the colour of sand after the sun begins to set, when its fading light smooths and darkens each grain, urging it to attain a new vibrancy. Every encounter with this kind of beauty seems an invitation to pain. Every such encounter leaves me disconsolate. I would have coped except that he looked at me after I danced with an intermittent yet persistent gaze, curious and youthful in a way that secures forgiveness with no questions asked. A strange and enigmatic look like the gaze of a sacred serpent that creates the world through the process of merely gazing at it, as if my body too, spent in dance, came into a new being through that gaze that I could not decipher but that I invited to burn through all my scars once more; a gaze through eyes rimmed as if with kohl and fringed with long, laughing lashes.

I danced without recorded music tonight—just the clapping of an audience that was enthusiastic and supportive as my hips cut through the space around me, inscribing yet again in small, sharp thrusts the lexicon of my hurting. And now I remain wide awake as if my body has resolved to carry out this vigil; a vigil strange and imposed, necessary and consuming. I danced without recorded music tonight—just rhythm that stirred my ghosts once more and now I await for them to complete their litany and retire so that the mourning inside can become, once more, imperceptible.

Cyprus: Various Mo(ve)ments

I want Cyprus to make sense to me as an imaginary erotic site. Why the obsession, you might wonder. The forces of conquest and domination (colonial, state, church and so on) must be understood as power relations that inscribe themselves on the body. Such power relations are what William Spurlin refers to when he argues that the sexual and struggles for erotic autonomy form significant axes of analysis (189). Moreover, dance and the erotic share one significant similarity: they are both endowed with "transformative powers" which, as Spurlin again notes (200), have been completely unrecognized by ideological analysts. The Cyprus Republic's anxious but insistent heterosexual posturing has obliterated the rights of sexual minorities and deferred necessary retheorizations of nation, citizenship, sexuality, and identity. At moments when these rights could not be obliterated, they were completely trivialized and mocked with self-righteousness. Heteronormativity, as a normalizing regime, perpetuates its ideological longevity sanctioned in its cause by the Republic.

Since the 1974 invasion of Cyprus by Turkish troops, the words "Den Xehno" (which literally translate into "I don't forget") have solidified into a ubiquitous slogan encountered everywhere from newspapers to self-adhesive stickers on car windows and shops. Unfortunately, the inflexible and ideological bias of this slogan has sought (and succeeded largely) to fixate Cypriot consciousness and has obliterated other narratives from surfacing and affecting in any substantial way the cultural and political landscape. In a strong sense, "Den Xehno" has been an attempt to dictate and control the subject's memory from within. The following three moments form part of anamnesiac practice that is, for me, a site of resistance and a subversion of the "Den xehno" slogan.

Mesaoria, 4 June 2003[5]

With Spurgeon Thompson, a friend and colleague, we are driving towards Famagusta to attend and present at a conference at the Eastern Mediterranean University. It is my first trip here after thirty years. In 1974, the border that divided the two parts of Cyprus was sealed with blood and destruction. Two months before I would not have been able to attend the conference, but because of the recent and somewhat unexpected development (the ease of restrictions in movement between the two parts of Cyprus) my participation at the event becomes a possibility. It is an overwhelming experience. The landscape speeds past us like a dream. The early morning light spreads across the Mesaoria plain gently urging the subtle and shifting hues of its stunning composition of rocks, plants, and earth to reveal themselves and begin their transformation. In my eager eyes, the earth seems abundant, fertile, and loving. As if the landscape conceals an oracle, I am begging it to speak, to narrate, and it indulges me—but only half-heartedly since it remains absorbed in its vibrant intercourse with the light. Mesaoria—with its old villages and river beds dense with eucalyptus, donkeys, and with the Pentadaktylos mountain range offering generously its imposing definition. I am thinking of Spivak again: the gaze I occupy has been inflected by my history. It is the sight/site into which I emerge and, although I do not want to privilege it, I do need to use it. How can I inhabit a different body and attempt another gaze? In the delirium that surrounds Cyprus's accession to the European Union, and the presumption of those Greek Cypriots who are keen to show off the official signature that confirms their European status, I insist on Mesaoria's non-Europeanness. I long to see its body as a confluence of narratives that reverberate across space and time, setting each Cypriot body into motion.

A Gym in Nicosia, September 2002

"Wa rimshi asmarani/Shabakna bil hawa" ("the eyelashes of the swarthy one/have entangled me in the nets of love").[6] Strangely, my focus on exercise allows me to observe people around me more accutely. Cypriot men must have the thickest and most languorous eyelashes I have ever set my hungry gaze upon; usually dark, playful, elongated, and entangled in their narcissistic self-absorption. Indifferent to the mechanical, often macho gym postures, eyelids indulge playfully and dance away with indifference. I relish the illicitness of such gazing at Cypriot male corporeality. In the teachings that we were meticulously indoctrinated by, hangings, killings, and beatings have been valorized and narrated endlessly as epics of remarkable adroitness and heroic national sacrifice. Purity of patriotic feeling in the midst of barbarity must, we learned, prevail over the anamnesis of contaminated passions and erotic possibilities.

Kalem Restaurant in Northern Nicosia, 17 August 2003

In an evening of speeches and performances that I organized jointly with Sylvia, my friend and belly dance teacher in Nicosia, I deliver a talk entitled "Dancing to the End of Love." Zehra, a new Cypriot friend from the Turkish side, is translating my words into Turkish. I use "dancing" in the title because I prefer the gerund form instead of the imperative "Dance

Me," with its suggestion of a partner (which I think Leonard Cohen has in mind for his song "Dance Me to the End of Love"). I am a solo dancer and any suggestion of leading a partner or being led freezes me completely. "Dancing to the End of Love" spins and undulates with a power that its unique grace breathes forth and plagues me with questions before, during, and after the event. In the emotional realm, where do we imagine that geographical point where Love ends? And how do we comprehend that space that dance traverses as it carries us with its flow to reach that place of ultimate fulfillment—that ecstatic telos where we consume the sacraments of desire and passion, in order to trans-form? And is the point of departure for this course always marked and accessible? Could we start from anywhere to "dance to the end of love" or does this place need designation? I also feel a strong connection between "dancing to the end of love" and memory—a certain nostalgia as if we have already been at this place but never truly experienced it. Dance is very much about finding a home. Perhaps not many people think about it in those terms but it certainly helps me when I do.

All this questioning and speculation do not make it to the talk. The moment at Kalem requires a delicate balancing between gentleness and pragmatism in dealing with the issues that the evening sets out to thematize. So, adorned and hip-scarfed, I am performing to "Oğlan, Oğlan," a tsifteteli sung in Turkish by Stelios Kazantzides, quite possibly the most beloved Greek male voice ever. I dance and play finger cymbals before an audience of Cypriots—Greek and Turkish. Abruptly, presumably because of some technical problem, the CD player stops but my audience continues to clap the rhythm and sing the lyrics in both the Cypriot dialects, urging me to continue dancing to their singing and clapping, and my finger cymbals. (What the Greek-Cypriots are singing is a familiar song that I have known but never thought of as the Greek version of "Oğlan, Oğlan," always considering it a different song.) It becomes a rare moment in this courtyard of a humble restaurant in old Nicosia—a performance that evokes a multitude of feelings, impulses, desires both for dancer and audience. In this constant shift between spaces and performances lie resistance and meanings, useful constructions and deconstructions. The recorded song then returns and blares through the loudspeakers, sounding distorted but dynamic, Kazantzides's voice a little clipped but completely new, as if the song has been given another birth.

As the curtain falls on my performance here, and separates me from my virtual audience, I will hurry backstage to change into other costumes, in those magical dressing rooms, which afford possibilities of see-ing and transformations, so that I prepare to go onstage yet again for the abuse and exaltation, disapprobation and trancing love which are evoked in my Cypriot drama.

Notes

Notes to Preface

1 By indicating her pronounciation of the term, I am attempting to relate the per-formativity of that particular exchange. In the manner that it was uttered, "Diskôrs" evoked the assumed gravity of her statements and rendering it here allows me to stage, so to speak, the moment for my reader.

2 I know only some details about his murder, yet researching the facts is obstructed by the complexity and sensitivity of the issue. Most likely because this narrative is the site of trauma, my mother is silent about it although occasionally she relates a few pieces of information. Interestingly, she believes that he was killed not by Turkish Cypriots but by nationalist Turks from Turkey who came to Cyprus to assist the Turkish Cypriot cause.

Notes to Chapter 1

1 Mariza Koch wrote the music based on a traditional tune and Michalis Fotiadis wrote the lyrics.

2 Mariza Koch, personal conversation, Thessaloniki, Greece, January 1991.

3 The lagouto is a string instrument whose name derives from the Arabic "al oud," which is also a popular musical instrument similar to the lagouto and also part of Greek folkloric tradition. For details on the history, playing, as well as making of the lagouto and the oud, see Phoivos Anoyiannakis's *Greek Folk Musical Instruments*, 210-54.

4 Although Greece's contribution to music, dance, and film (to cite only a few examples of artistic output in Greece) is extremely valuable on a global level, this contribution reifies only in the artistic taste and, quite often, memory of those who follow and are affected by Greek culture. For example, the immensely rich library of the Greek Television archives—nothing less than a national treasure of inter-national importance—lacks proper care and adequate cataloguing. Although such material disregard could be signs of a lingering oral tradition, the exigencies of a technologically dependant world are interfering with memory and its construc-tion of reality, thus making material archives and the emergence of a new cultural historiography of Greece increasingly necessary. Such development would also assist in making the practice of documenting, scripting, and theorizing culture more strongly rooted in the Greek world.

5 In his book *Ο Κόσμος του Ελληνικού Χορού* [*The World of Hellenic Dance*] Alkis Raftis offers an interesting, albeit simple, definition of "traditional" that seems relevant to the argument I am trying to make here. For Raftis "traditional" refers to those parts of cultural instruction that are bequeathed by one generation to the next and continue to play an organic role in their environment. A dance, for example, that has been taught by the parents to their children who perform it at a village celebration is traditional. A routine taught by a dance teacher in an urban setting does not qualify as traditional dance. In my argument about the Eurovision contest, I suggest that the incorporation of the lagouto into the 1976 presentation had a traditional character and function. What varies is that this traditionality was transposed to a world stage.

6 *Zorba the Greek* and *Never on Sunday* were two films whose enormous international success contributed greatly to the popularization of the bouzouki. Mikis Theodorakis and Manos Hadjidakis respectively composed the musical scores for the two films and relied heavily on the bouzouki to lend that particular musical colour and texture that people around the world came to recognize and associate with "Greece."

7 In fact, these signifiers, the lagouto and its player and Mariza in her black dress, were somewhat disturbing in the context of contest politics. The emphasis of the event needed to be on songs that qualified as "European" not only in terms of Western musical scales but also in terms of texture. Songs were to disregard, as much as possible, the distinct characteristics of specific regional traditions.

8 In 1976, for example, the British pop group Brotherhood of Man won the contest with an uninspiring ditty entitled "Save All Your Kisses for Me." This song, juxtaposed with Koch's lament for the tragedy of war in Cyprus, forms a perfect illustration of my point about tedious artistic output that meets with success and recognition while it buries critique and any useful meanings.

9 Especially during the censorious years of the military dictatorship (1967-1974), folk songs were employed to promote an exoticized, quaint vision of Greece in the domestic and international sphere with the goal of attracting Western tourism. In chapter 5 I will discuss the interventions in folk tradition in detail, yet what I want to say here is that in the midst of this cultural revision, Mariza Koch performed well-known folk songs from various regions of Greece solely with percussive accompaniment, thus rendering tradition using an avant-garde musical technique. Her intervention signalled an artistic resistance to the oppressive regime of the colonels. Her interpretations performed a necessary violation of the idyllic picturesqueness of the Greek countryside, which lost its "innocence" and "quaintness" in the uncompromising and hard sound of drums and bongos. Meanwhile, the traditional derivation of the lyrics in her albums of the early 1970s made it impossible for the Junta censors to censor the songs.

10 Although Koestenbaum speaks of opera, his description of its effects resembles my own experience of Mariza Koch. He says: "I'm a lemming, imprinted by the soprano, my existence an after effect of her crescendo. Straight socialization makes queer people discard their bodies, listening restores queer embodiment, if only for the duration of a phrase. Forceful displays of singing insist that the diva has a body and so do you because your heartbeat shifts in uncanny affinity with her ascent" (42).

11 Mariza Koch combined a presence and a musical temperament that determined her original trajectory in Greek musical culture. Her mixed parentage—a Greek

mother and a German father (hence her surname)—bequeathed physical characteristics that would place her more readily in Northwestern Europe than in Greece. Her straight and very long, blonde hair has given her a dramatic appeal and enhanced her performative potential. At the same time, her temperament and repertoire have been distinctly Greek. As a young boy, I was mystified by her features and made her the closest to a diva that a queer boy in the West would admire.

12 I place "queerly" in scare quotes for two reasons. I am introducing it into a context (the Cyprus of my childhood) where it had no designated space, no existence, and where I certainly had no awareness of it and, secondly, I want to mark the anachronistic employment of the term.

13 "Cypriotness" is a vague, shifting term whose political interpretations vary enormously even among those prepared to identify as "Greek Cypriot." Investigating the construction of ethnic identity among elementary school children in the Greek part of the island, Spyros Spyrou observes that the indexes of "Greekness" and "Cypriotness" vary greatly according to political, class, and ideological affiliation. "In practice, there are multiple constructions of identity claimed by different groups who situate themselves variously in the ideological space between [the Hellenocentric and Cypriocentric] poles ... Culture or identity, in this particular sense, is more akin to what Verderey (1994) called a 'zone of *disagreement* and *contest* rather than 'a zone of shared meanings'" (171). As dominant ideology, though, Greek Cypriot nationalism deploys certain markers that are clear and recognizable by Greek Cypriots.

14 While I find Herzfeld's assessment of the Greek predicament useful, I am rather uneasy with his implicit assumption that all Greeks share a single "nativist" ideology—an assumption that, apart from being Romantic, might also be imprecise.

15 Kamboureli questions the mode of self-identification in criticism. She resists the pressure to position ourselves in our work, a pressure which, at times, assumes the force of a political imperative in the arena of critical debates. For Kamboureli, the problematics of such positioning stem from "the disciplinary, hence totalizing, intent that informs the gestures of self-location [that] might be seen as an instance of restricted economy, a closed system of relations that articulates events in regulated ways while remaining unaware of the effects of its control" (5).

16 In her introduction to *Tango and the Political Economy of Passion*, Savigliano elaborates on these "voices" in a way that I can identify—with some adjustments, of course, since Savigliano writes from a female perspective and a Latino background. "In writing this book," she says, "I have dealt with many conflicting voices: academized and poetic, orderly and chaotic, male-hegemonic and female-subversive, elitist and impoverished, collective and personal, totalizing and specific, deconstructed and reconstructive, white and mestizo, pragmatic and nostalgic, in English and in Spanish ... of the colonizer and of the colonized" (4). (In my case, it would not be English and Spanish but English and Greek and the Cypriot dialect.)

17 In this article, Sellers-Young attempts a clear analysis of the dance's acculturation in North America. However, she refers to the dance as "Islamic," a term that I resist since I find the dance extends beyond Islam, geographically and culturally.

18 In an interesting article, Richard Phillips argues that Burton employed travel geography as an enabling point of departure rather than an end in itself. Although pederasty threatens constantly to transcend its precisely defined zone, Burton's geographical containment of it seems to define it as a discrete, containable form of sexuality. Ultimately, however, Phillips believes that Burton's "pornotopia" protests against Victorian homophobia. "[Burton] charts sexual geography that seems, on first inspection, to be rigid, static and divided, but turns out to be fluid, open-ended and integrated" (85).

19 In John Scagliotti's documentary *Dangerous Living: Coming Out in the Developing World* a number of interviewees from parts of the so-called "developing world" affirm that the sanctioned homophobia and persistent persecution against alternative sexualities in their countries are the product of colonialism. Adnan Ali, a gay man from Pakistan who currently lives in London, England, says that in Pakistan the law against homosexuality is not a *sharia* (religious) law but an inheritance from his country's colonial past. Moreover, Rodney Lutalo from Uganda (currently under asylum in Canada) and Anna Leah Sarabia from the Philippines also voice their belief that, contrary to the authorities' propaganda in their countries, it is not homosexuality that is a Western phenomenon but homophobia. "The British introduced homophobia into Uganda," Lutalo says, "and when they left they forgot to erase that." See also the transcript of the interviews from *Dangerous Living* at <www.afterstonewall.com>.

20 In her notes to the "Introduction" of *Between Men*, Sedgwick problematizes the term "homophobia," which she finds "fraught with difficulties." She agrees, however, that "the ideological and thematic treatments of male homosexuality to be discussed from the late eighteenth century onward do combine fear and hatred in a way that is appropriately called phobic" (219). Byrne Fone is also skeptical about the term which he finds inadequate for the multitude of locutions that homosexual disapprobation includes. Homophobia, he writes, "is even more recently invented than 'homosexual' and its precision and accuracy are still open to question. It is not satisfactory, constructed as it is from a slang abbreviation for 'homosexual' joined with *phobia*, which means fear but not dislike. For lack of a better term, I will use it, usually anachronistically, to name what I look for in history" (424, n5). What is particularly interesting for me is to observe its tentative and unconvincing entry into the Greek vocabulary of Cyprus where the scene of sexual behaviour is still dominated by an intriguing combination of "older" perceptions of sex (and I am thinking here of the distinction between the sexual act versus the sexual identity, a distinction that allows many heterosexually identified men to have sex with other men by taking only the active part) and more recent modes of understanding sex as a mutual act where the axis of separation is not between passive and active roles but sexual identification, that is homo/heterosexual. In identifying "older" and "more recent" modes of perceiving sex, I do not wish to stress some linearity in sexual politics development; rather I want to draw attention to recent trends in globalization of sexualities. In order to assist my thinking about the issue, I list these two modes, very crudely, as precolonial and postcolonial acts of love.

21 The British were not the only Western Europeans anxious to establish these diachronic connections. The German Magda Ohnefalsch-Richter, wife of the famous archaeologist Max Ohnefalsch-Richter, lived in Cyprus with her hus-

band between 1894 and 1913. Her study of life on the island yielded the project *Griechische Sitten und Gebräuche auf Cypern* [*Greek Customs and Traditions of Cyprus*] where she delights in delineating all that she finds connecting the modern inhabitants of the island to their classical ancestors. A Greek translation of her book has been published by the Cyprus Popular Bank Cultural Centre. Interestingly, but not surprisingly, powerful financial institutions of the island and government presses are keen on publishing Western Europeans' research on topics such as customs, antiquity, and the Greekness of Cyprus, since these Europeans' discourse has formed part of the dominant rhetoric and has also seen a rigorous application in the founding of the allegiances of the modern Cyprus republic.

22 In his article "Those on the Other Side," Spyrou also states that "it was under the British that the two communities developed their respective nationalisms that symbolically anchored their identities to Greece and Turkey respectively" (169-70).

23 Among the points that Makarios Drousiotis makes is that the Turkish Cypriots were not the only people excluded from EOKA (Hellenic Association of Cypriot Fighters). Members of AKEL, the communist party, were also expressly forbidden from joining the ranks of Cypriot fighters (74). This could be an indication that Western (mainly British) interests regulated the course and character of the uprising. Although it may seem absurd that Britain would orchestrate an uprising against its own administration, the possibility of British involvement or, at least, British consent, is now discussed by various historians and journalists including Drousiotis in *EOKA: The Obscure Side*.

24 Greece as the cradle of Western Europe involves a long process of conceptualization that Martin Bernal examines as the "Aryan Model" in his study *Black Athena*. The book raised controversy because it challenged hitherto accepted notions of the origins of Western Civilization in Ancient Greece and exposed the racism and "continental chauvinism" (2) of historiography that persistently denied the possible influence of African and Semitic cultures on classical civilization.

25 Research priorities and publications in Cyprus focus on the "national problem" (the 1974 invasion by Turkish troops and the continuing occupation of the northern part of the island) and not on a critique of recent historical events. In other words, the favourite topic is not "what is our share of the responsibility" but, rather, "how beautiful is our island and look what they have done to us." Government and church scholarships usually encourage projects that recreate, on the one hand, the island as picturesque and replete with archaeological monuments, and as martyred land on the other. Certainly, the role of the upper-class Greeks in the Greek-Turkish conflict would not make an agreeable topic.

26 Like most men of his generation and class (he was a farmer), my grandfather had no formal education. The Greek Cypriot dialect is oral and contains sounds that the Greek alphabet does not represent. The institution of public education with its aspiration to "modernize" the Cypriot citizen brought about the demise of the Cypriot dialect, since the emphasis was on "proper" Greek as opposed to the vernacular with its strong Turkish (but also English) linguistic influence.

27 For a spirited and engaging analysis of the moustache and its important iconic implications in performing masculinity in Middle Eastern societies, see Hassan Daoud's essay "Those Two Heavy Wings of Manhood: On Moustaches" in *Imagined Masculinities*, 273-80.

28 "Economy" as a theoretical term has been in vogue for awhile—a trend that I find entirely agreeable, even though my talent in economics is embarrassingly inadequate. As I understand it, the term denotes a system with an often emotional currency and with exchanges happening on various fronts. Marta Savigliano, of course, has deployed the term in ways that have endowed it with fresh significance. Also noteworthy is Mary Louise Pratt's notion of a "contact zone" which is the medium where "economies" enact their most intriguing shapes.

29 Initially, my intention was to italicize these sections. In a workshop given at the University of Calgary in the fall of 1999, Susan Foster suggested such an approach in writing about dance. For the finished product of such an attempt see the "Introduction" to *Corporealities: Dancing Knowledge, Culture and Power,* where a variety of fonts and styles represents each contributor to the volume, making up a choreographed verbal inscription. Because the various contributions are distinguished typographically, this particular introduction has the look and feel of a performance where each contributor enters, dances/speaks solo or in dialectic with another contributor, and then exits. However, my sections did not work in an italicized form, either because during the years of acquiring English as a second language I assimilated only a stringent version of it, or because I lack practice and, therefore, virtuosity in directing such ambitious attempts.

30 Regarding the terms East and West, I am fully conscious that more often than not they form generalizations that may detract from the specificity of the arguments that I formulate. Nevertheless, I persist in their use because, as Joseph Boone points out, in a discussion involving West and East it is impossible not to generalize at times. Moreover, in certain contexts, Boone, uses these "rhetorical markers as shorthand for much more complex geographic and psychological realities" (70-1, n1).

31 I have reservations regarding Bartholdy's assumption on the ethnicity of the *koçek.* In a civilization as complex and cosmopolitan (meaning an exchange of many different cultures) as the Ottoman Empire, one cannot pretend to make accurate assessments of the culture following even a lengthy visit.

32 Leona Wood, from the booklet accompanying the album *Music of the Ghawazee.* Wood cites Raafat Nasser-Eddin as her consultant on this point. The album consists of live recordings made by Aisha Ali at Thebes, Egypt.

33 See Alain Weber's liner notes for *Egypt: Music of the Nile from the Desert to the Sea* (18). Because of their relevance to my discussion here, I provide a full paragraph of Weber's statements on the *awâlim:* "The legendary and fascinating almées (almée or âlima, from the Arab 'elm,' or 'knowledge,' referring to those who possess musical knowledge) were formerly professional singers. Serving as living repositories of the ancient qayna, the slave-singers of pre-Islamic times, when they filled the sultans' courts, the almées were doubly penalized: as women; and as musicians. Exiled to far-flung villages, they performed at wedding feasts, singing songs that were often erotic, crude, and subjective and that also recalled the performances of the ghâwazi, dancers from the nawar or balhâwanat gypsy clans exiled to Upper Egypt by Muhammad Álî."

34 The annotations by Lane, Burton, and Torrens that I use here are provided in a two-volume edition entitled *The Arabian Nights Entertainments.* This edition features Richard Burton's translation but all three translators' notes appear in a "Supplement" at the end of each volume with pagination beginning at 1 in each

supplement. The full, lengthy title of this collection indicates clearly its character and scope: *The Arabian Nights Entertainments containing sixty-five stories told by Shahrazade the Sultaness to divert Shahryar the Sultan from the execution of a vow he had made to avenge the disloyalty of his first Sultaness; and containing a better account of the customs, manners and religion of the Eastern nations than is to be met with in any edition hitherto published; because the text is one which Sir Richard Burton himself desired to own: the definitive and all-inclusive Burton translation with the addition of the notes upon the text prepared by those scholars who had previously translated the text into English from the Arabic, notably Henry Torrens and Edward Lane and John Payne; and it is embellished with miniature paintings made by Arthur Szyk for the Heritage Press, New York.* Notes by different annotators on the same textual point retain the same numerical designation throughout the discussion in the "Supplements." I use only Volume 1.

35 In a prefatory note to this two-volume edition of the *Arabian Nights Entertainments* John Winterich points out that "something of the character of each translator and annotator will emerge in reading the notes … The reader will find these four personalities emerging as clearly as if a photographer were developing portrait negatives whereof the lineaments of the subjects gradually but unmistakably come into view" (viii).

36 In his notes, Burton makes an interesting comparison between made-up eyes and miners fresh from the colliery. This comparison, which falls squarely in the premise of Ann McClintock's exploration of the domestic and exotic spheres, illustrates the ways in which working-class British people were portrayed in relation to Oriental people: "Moslems in Central Africa apply Kohl not to the thickness of the eyelid but upon both outer lids, fixing it with some greasy substance. The peculiar Egyptian (and Syrian) eye with its thick fringes of jet-black lashes, looking like lines of black drawn with soot, easily suggests the simile. In England I have seen the same appearance amongst miners fresh from the colliery" ("Supplement" 13, n21). The association here is interesting because the miners on the job are in a sense enslaved in an underground setting while the Egyptians or Syrians have a similar look but are not working in subterranean galleries. The comparison is an effort to equate an artistic practice with the plight of a large group of working-class people (who after all fuel the economy of Britain) and, second, it reveals, I think, an erotic interest in both the made-up "Orientals" and in the miners whose faces show work toil, that Burton may have found sexy, as well as affinities with other abject people, most likely female.

37 The last week of April 2003 marked a crucial development in the history of the island. At this time, the Turkish-Cypriot leader Rauf Denktash decided to open the border and allow people living in the North and South to cross the line of separation with certain restrictions. This is an overwhelming development that could form the initial stages of finding a solution to the division. Nonetheless, the full implications of this movement between the North and South by Turkish and Greek-Cypriots respectively have yet to be realized. For a detailed discussion of this development, see the article "Cyprus after History," by Spurgeon Thompson, Stavros Stavrou Karayanni, and Myria Vassiliadou in *Interventions: International Journal of Postcolonial Studies* 6.2 (June 2004): 282-99.

Notes to Chapter 2

1 The spelling of the name Kuchuk Hanem enjoys a large range of variations even within Steegmuller's various publications and editions of Flaubert's letters and travel memoirs. In what reads almost like an aside to a discussion about the trope of descent used by Flaubert to represent Oriental women, Lisa Lowe theorizes the diversity in transliteration: "like the name Kuchuk-Hânem, which occurs inconsistently in *Voyage* and *Correspondence*—appearing as Ruchuk-Hânem, Ruchiouck-Hânem, and then Kuchuk-Hânem, as if, despite anxious repetition to ensure its fixity, the name can never be arrested in an identical form—the topos of the descending oriental woman is repeated variously, with different nuances, different emphases" (87).

2 In *Beyond the Veil*, Mernissi's discussion focuses on twentieth-century developments in mostly Arab countries. Moreover, Kathleen Fraser, who has researched women's position in Muslim societies, has found that Islamic Egypt allowed many lower-class Egyptian women to have their own female trades which they pursued actively for monetary gain. Fraser's research is still unpublished. I owe this information to personal communication with her.

3 Parts of this passage combined with selections from Flaubert on Kuchuk Hanem and Azizeh form the verbal narrative that accompanies the choreodrama "Dancing Girls" from *Arabic Dance in Performance*, which Wendy Buonaventura composed and performed with Jacqueline Jamal in 1998 (Videotape, Cinnabar Productions).

4 It seems to me quite striking and noteworthy that George W. Curtis's description of Kuchuk's choreography here is markedly different from more recent ghawazee dances as filmed by Aisha Ali in Upper Egypt. In her documentary *Dances of Egypt* there is extensive footage of the Banaat Mazin of Luxor, a group of sisters who performed professionally through the 1970s and the '80s. They were, apparently, the most famous ghawazee of recent times and made their father wealthy with the income he amassed from their dancing. Ali's footage is from the mid-1970s. Kuchuk Hanem's dancing as interpreted by Curtis displays some of the dramatic quality that Oriental dance has today making researchers, dancers, and musicians speculate about the character of ghawazee performance in the Upper Egypt of the mid-nineteenth century.

5 The most famous performer whose choreography typically evolved not across space but in a vertical and horizontal corporeal axis was the revered Tahia Carioca. Because of her ability to dance covering very limited space, she was popularly said to "dance on a single tile," thus the title of Linda Swanson's multi-media presentation "They Said She Could Dance on a Single Tile."

6 Ahmad is helpful in identifying some of the weaknesses and lapses of Said's *Orientalism*. Nevertheless, Ahmad's critique cannot diminish the possibilities that Said's argument has offered. Using Foucault's theory, Said created a language and an approach that launched the field of postcolonial studies. His work has made an enormous contribution to the theorizing of the colonialist project and the colonial condition. Although Robert Young accepts Ahmad's criticisms, he feels "it could also be argued that they also involve a form of category mistake: the investigation of the discursive construction of colonialism does not seek to replace or exclude other forms of analysis, whether they be historical, geographical, economic, military, or political" (*Colonial Desire* 163).

7   Edward Said did not resist the challenge of writing about movement in dance throughout his writing career. Long after the publication of *Orientalism*, Said wrote about Tahia Carioca and expatiated on her dance style in evocative language. Said admits that this celebrated dancer's performances formed "a rich but relatively unexplored memory" ("Homage to a Belly-Dancer" 354). Said marked Carioca's passing in 1999 with another article entitled "Farewell to Tahia."

8   Constantinople is now widely known as Istanbul. This is the ancient city that Constantine renamed after himself and made the capital of Byzantium in 324 AD. Both names (the modern Istanbul and the Byzantine Constantinople) derive from Greek, Constantinople meaning "City of Constantine" and "Istanbul" being a corrupt version of the phrase "To the City" (Eis tin Polin). It is interesting to note that during the Ottoman Empire the city continued to be called Constantinople. Its name was changed to Istanbul in 1930 under the sway of Turkish nationalism (initiated by Kemal Ataturk). Constantinople continues to house what is known as Ecumenical Patriarchate, the seat of Greek Orthodox faith. Greek speakers often do not like to use "Istanbul," which they consider a corrupt form of a Greek phrase and a sign of Turkish nationalism. In this book, I use Constantinople also because this is how the city is named in the travel narratives that I discuss. I thank Athanasios Tavouktsoglou for providing much of the information in this note and for alerting me to the sensitive politics behind the naming of this city.

9   Andrea Deagon suggests that Flaubert's derogatory references to Kuchuk's bad tooth and the ugliness of some of the dancers—Hassan el-Balbeissi, for example, whom I will discuss in the following chapter—are "a flippant articulation of his perception of a real aesthetic difference between the conventions of performance of his culture and the East: that in Egypt, idiosyncrasies and flaws did not negate the charm, ability and success of these 'ugly' yet strangely beautiful performers" ("The Image of the Eastern Dancer" 14).

10 On this theme see especially "Introductions" and "Chapter 5: Exotic Encounters" in Marta Savigliano's *Tango and the Political Economy of Passion*.

11 This image refers to the tale of Saint George who killed the terrible dragon (whose menace and torture afflicted the whole land) and married the beautiful and chaste princess. The slaying of the dragon is a very popular theme in Christian, especially Orthodox, iconography, and even though there is no immediate reference to any marriage in Curtis's narrative, the image is appropriate because it combines religion with male virtue and valour. Because religion often becomes a coercive instrument in the hands of despotic men who implement measures for moral control, the image of Curtis as St. George is a comment on the endorsement of hegemonic values by an imperial subject and the self-righteousness that accompanies the act.

12 Despite what I suggest about Curtis and his response to the moral threat embedded in Kuchuk and her dancers, his narrative did generate discomfort and even offence. Paul Eugene Monty found that *Nile Notes* received fairly favourable reviews in England and the United States, yet the passages on the "dancing girls of Egypt … were in some quarters held to be reprehensible" (127-28).

13 In contrast, Kuchuk also supplies an apex in Flaubert and Colet's love relationship and its crises as I discuss earlier. In this latter case, Lisa Lowe's argument is very insightful: "in constructing women as machines, however, Flaubert makes

Colet (as addressee, as witness) complicit in her own degradation as a woman, an uneasy accomplice to his exploitation of Kuchuk-Hanem" (76-77, n1).

Notes to Chapter 3

1 Paying particular attention to the visual arts, Wijdan Ali discusses the impact of Mohamed Ali's artistic reformations in Egypt in his article "Modern Painting in the Mashriq": "when Mohamed Ali became Egypt's effective ruler in 1805, after breaking away from Ottoman authority, he introduced European aesthetics to the urban Egyptian intellectual milieu. He displayed interest in the arts as well as sciences and military skills, and sent several study missions to Europe, which concentrated on learning the arts of engraving, painting, and sculpture, among other subjects. These individuals taught at technical craft schools once they returned" (364). The teaching of artistic skill imported from elsewhere sees a parallel with the projects of the Tunisian National Folkloric Troupe as filmed and discussed by Aisha Ali in her documentary *Dances of North Africa—Volume 1: Morocco and Tunisia*. While filming dance drills by the troupe's members, Ali observes that the men's movements—which I find impressive and compelling—are less traditional (as she puts it) than the women's because their leaders had been sent to Romania to study choreographic techniques. Romania may not carry the imperial prestige of Western Europe, yet in both cases, Mohamed Ali's artistic reforms in the early nineteenth century and the Tunisian National Folkloric Troupe's choreographies in the mid 1970s, there is an interesting connection that underscores the constantly evolving condition of art and its ideological as well as artistic implications. Moreover, the men's dance technique and Aisha Ali's comment on it suggest an intriguing intervention that challenges notions of purity, authenticity, fixity, and continuity that hold such powerful sway in the perception of "Oriental" traditions (a perception that Aisha Ali herself champions as a valuable quality of her film projects).

2 Sophie Lane-Poole, Edward Lane's sister, visited Egypt in 1842 with her famous brother and attended the royal wedding of Muhammad Ali's daughter Zaynab. Lane-Poole recorded her observations of the wedding in great detail. Apparently, singing and dancing were such significant parts of the ceremony that performances lasted entire days for a whole week. One of the conclusions that Kathleen Fraser reaches from Lane-Poole's narrative is that there is evidence to assume the existence of "a recognized and widely accepted dance aesthetic … in mid-nineteenth century Egypt at all levels" ("Public and Private Entertainment" 37).

3 At this point Berger quotes a section from the same passage from Vivant Denon (205), that I quote in my epigraph to this chapter. Berger, however, cites the wrong page for the quotation.

4 Particularly relevant here are Anthony Shay's comments in "The Male Dancer." Shay comments on Wendy Buonaventura's description of belly dance as a female form of cultural expression: "feminists who have adopted belly dance as an emblem of the female sexual revolution in the 1970s often revel in romanticized descriptions of belly dance as a female form of cultural expression" (14).

5 Andrea Deagon explores the opposing views of belly dance within feminist discourse in "Feminism and Belly Dance." Exploring the tensions between female objectification on the one hand, and empowerment on the other, Deagon poses

the question: "Is belly dance really empowering for women, or does it simply bring 'women as sex objects' into a different range of venues than before?" (10). In response, Deagon sensitively balances these delicate issues, discussing realms of feminist enquiry that are pertinent to belly dancers: ownership of women's sexuality within patriarchy, Sartre's notion of "bad faith," and essentialism (10).

6   In *Critical Terrains*, Lisa Lowe demonstrates, quite successfully I find, that Lady Mary Wortley Montagu's observations on Turkish culture and society are governed by profound paradoxes. Her writings are marked by what Lowe calls, "multivalence." While on the one hand, Montague redresses many of what she insists are the misconceptions and inaccurate representations of Turkish women, propagated by male travel writers, some of her descriptions "resonate with traditional occidental imaginings of the Orient as exotic, ornate, and mysterious, imaginary qualities fundamental to eighteenth-century Anglo-Turkish relations" (31).

7   Here I quote Andrea Deagon's translation of Martial's passage from her article "Framing the Ancient History of Oriental Dance" (38). This article is significant in offering a rare reading of Martial's epigrams with brief references to dances that are discussed in some detail, drawing insightful inferences about the dancers and their art in the latter years of the Roman Empire.

8   Metin And quotes an omitted paragraph from Dr. Covel's published diaries (the manuscript is in the British Museum) that describes a sequence of "little plays or interludes, all using the most beastly brutish language possible." These interludes represented "the damnable act of buggery in the grossest manner possible, with men, boys and beasts, whereof in show came in many…acting upon all fours" (149).

9   Hamilton's book is a compilation of various travellers' accounts that she does not always cite in any detail. Although she is supposedly concerned with customs and ceremonies from the entire universe, a truly overwhelming and ambitious task, her emphasis is on sexual intrigue, scandal, and gossip from what in her day was termed "the Orient." In recent times, authors such as Carla Coco have emulated Hamilton's project. Limiting her focus to the Ottoman Empire (as opposed to Hamilton's "universe"), Coco attempts a very similar task in *Secrets of the Harem*, a lavish and extravagantly illustrated volume whose sole service, it seems, is to underpin the lasting appeal of the Orientalist fantasy and the harem in particular.

10 Özdemir's willingness to address openly the sexuality of the dance and offer an account that is less puritan than what one often encounters is refreshing. But, the package he offers does not seem intended to reform our viewing of the dance and open up possibilities of embracing homo- and hetero-eroticism as forms of vital artistic expression. Rather, his text and photographs seem to be geared towards a heterosexist aesthetic and intended, almost exclusively, for straight male consumption.

11 See Letter to Bouilhet, "Between Girga and Assiut, June 2, 1850" in *Letters* (121), and *Flaubert in Egypt* (203-204). In the latter source, Steegmuller provides an informative footnote on Jean-Paul Sartre's disbelief that Flaubert consummated homosexual experiences in the baths. Steegmuller writes: "in [Sartre's] opinion, all Flaubert's pederastic talk in his letters to Louis Bouilhet is merely a form of joking, common between him and his friends; there were no homosexual relations between them as some have thought; and all the references to bardashes in the

baths were the swank of a traveler wanting to impress a stay-at-home with his exotic experiences" (204). In order to support his position, Sartre offers to analyze various pieces of evidence, though I find that what is needed is not merely evidence testifying to the "truth" of Flaubert's sexual escapades on tour. What interests me is the theoretical implications behind the imperative of such narratives and what meanings these various reconstructions of a famous, allegedly straight man's sexual behaviour offer.

12 Pothos is a Greek term for desire. I prefer to use it here because for me the Greek term signifies a stronger and more fervent attraction towards that which generates longing.

13 Byrne Fone's work has offered a very elaborate development of Ramsay Burt's comment. Fone's *Homophobia: A History* is an ambitious and significant historical survey that demonstrates the various forms that homophobia has taken from classical Greece to the present. Most importantly, the book investigates the injuctions of religion, government, law, and science over same-sex sexual practice during various periods, and the consequences of these injunctions.

14 Fifi Abdou's interpretations are at times so sexually explicit that for some critics her artistic accomplishments achieve little else than confirm her status as a disreputable dancer. Such a notion holds such sway that I suspect that Edward Said has in mind, among many others, Fifi Abdou when he contrasts Tahia Carioca's talent with lesser dancers: "that smile has seemed to me symbolic of Tahia's distinction in a culture that featured dozens of dancers called Zouzou and Fifi, most of them treated as barely a notch above prostitutes" ("Homage to a Belly-Dancer" 349).

Notes to Chapter 4

1 This was not all the disruption that Salomé and her decadent male disciples were capable of. Showalter informs us that this subversive gang threatened the all-important class boundaries: "In terms of class, too, the new woman and the decadent seemed to violate proper hierarchies and social organisms. The transgression of class boundaries in their fiction gave rise to great alarm; both celebrated romantic alliances between the classes, with both men and women turning to working class lovers for a passion and tenderness missing in their own class surroundings" (169).

2 The pseudonym "Little Egypt" was given to one of the performers at the 1893 Chicago World Exposition. Her figure has sparked a great deal of interest and speculation to the point that it has become lore in the world of Middle Eastern dance. Donna Carlton's *Looking for Little Egypt* undertakes to unravel the mystery of this dancer's identity and assess the importance of her role in transmitting this particular dance tradition to North America.

3 Despite this negotiation on Allan's part, her tour to India had to be banned because "imperial values imagined that Maud's erotic dance would excite the 'rich native' to an unsafe degree" (Hoare 87).

1 In making this comment I am echoing Inderpal Grewal: "The education of the working class by means of institutions such as the British Museum and the department stores continued and furthered the rise of imperialism, another function of nationalism" (128).

2 Although lacking in focus and rather general in its approach, Raftis's book presents one of the few instances where the myth of classical continuity in Greek dance is challenged. He opens the chapter "Dance in Ancient Greece" as follows: "Every writer who deals with the dances of modern Greece considers it his obligation to assert that they are the same as the dances of the Greeks of antiquity. Accordingly, he may provide a phrase from an ancient text, or a picture from some ancient pottery as strong proof of the continuity of the race, as if proof is necessary. Such naïve treatment covers with a dose of facile patriotism the nonexistence of serious study on modern Greek dance" (my translation, 22). Raftis's argument is important but remains undeveloped in his book. It is an argument that has informed my own position and has become fundamental to this chapter on Hellenism and Greek dance.

3 In an attempt to offer some background information on Ali Pasha, Leslie A. Marchand, the editor of Byron's diaries, provides two footnotes that are drenched in exotica and gothic aura (apart from the brief biographical details): "Ali Pasha (1741-1822) was born at Tepelene in Albania.... When Byron arrived, he had made himself despotic ruler of the whole of what is now modern Greece as far south as the Gulf of Corinth, and of parts of Albania. He had subdued or driven out by treachery the Suliotes, who long defied him, and he used rivals to his advantage, including the French and English in the Ionian islands. By cunning, treachery, and the use of bandits as soldiers when it suited him, he had raised himself from a petty leader of robber bands to a ruler more powerful in his own domains than the Sultan himself.... He was short and fat and had a long white beard, and looked benign. But stories of his barbaric cruelty to enemies were well known ... Veli Pasha, Ali's second son, was master of the Morea (Peloponnesus). Both father and son had a penchant for young boys, and Veli's treachery, cruelty, and lasciviousness exceeded even those of his father" (vol. I, 226, n1-2). Such juxtaposition of abstract nouns and adjectives strays from Marchand's nominal purpose in the footnotes (to explain and elaborate on the historical aspect of Byron's journals), and fulfils an appetite for Oriental decadence. Apart from pederasty, also noteworthy is the trope of the Eastern son-in-office who emulates the father's ruthlessness, cruelty, and sexual excesses, a trope favoured by Occidental sensibility because it afforded Western "civilization" and "progress" added poignancy in their sanctimonious pose. Indeed, such Orientalist depiction of this Ottoman ruler and his son is more in tune with translations of the *Arabian Nights* than the kind of document that Marchand is producing.

4 See Louis Crompton *Byron and Greek Love* for a detailed discussion of Byron's travels to Greece and his motivations in leaving England. Crompton identifies Georgian homophobia as a primary cause for Byron's longing for an extended stay in Greece. His study remains the most influential and thorough treatment of the subject to date.

Stathis Gourgouris makes the interesting assertion that Byron inevitably turns into the "Philhellenic commodity" when he "becomes himself the object of the gaze—as if the gaze flies through the air like a boomerang—which is tantamount to saying that he falls right into the abyss of his own field of vision" (137-38). What remains unspoken in Gourgouris's analysis is that it was Byron's queer desires that opened the chasm that ultimately consumed Byron.

5   A common problem with transliteration of terms foreign to English is the discrepancies in the English spelling of the same foreign term. Even the same author, for example, may change the spelling of a transliterated term. *Ρεμπέτικα*, for example, is spelled *rembetika* by Gail Holst in her book *Road to Rembetika*, while in an article she published in 1998 she spells it *rebetika*.

6   In her article, Caterina Pizanias describes Stratou as "a ballet dancer in the mould of Martha Graham and Isadora Duncan, with impeccable conservative credentials" (26). Pizanias's information seems to be erroneous since no other evidence shows Stratou to be a dancer in any tradition. In her memoirs, *A Tradition, An Adventure* (Μία Παράδοση, Μία Περιπέτεια), Stratou mentions studies in theatre, her talent in music, and her gift in singing, but nowhere does she mention studies in dance. In fact, while in Athens conducting research on the Dora Stratou Greek Dance Theatre, Anthony Shay was informed by dancers and by Alkis Raftis, the new director of the theatre, that Dora Stratou could not dance a step. According to Shay, it would seem that Stratou was also incapable of conducting research (*Choreographic Politics* 262-63).

7   Some interesting details concerning Stratou's temperament and conduct emerge from the interviews that Anthony Shay conducted in Athens among members of her dance company. An anonymous informant says she was "authoritative and vulgar and ran the company with an iron hand. She knew nothing of folklore and could not dance. She used the threat of firing company members at a time when unemployment was so high in Greece that no one dared cross her. While touring in Switzerland, ten company members defected. Stratou was so enraged she called the Swiss authorities and had the unfortunate members deported" (265). I find these details relevant since they suggest an abusive and relentless despot rather than a "rescuer" of folklore. What she could not persuade, she would inflict and impose. Such mode of action is characteristic of the authoritative nature of her claims, while the austerity with which she imposed those claims at all costs certainly relies on a kind of hegemonic assumption.

8   A quotation from Vigarello in Savigliano articulates a similar concept in the context of court society dance: "Dancing was to be practiced with a great deal of caution, as it threatened to become 'dirty and immodest,' and to go beyond all degrees of propriety. Dancing must be the restrainer of passions [fear, melancholia, rage and joy].… From that point on, dance inevitably appeared full of contradictions" (249).

9   For a full discussion of these issues, see my review of Anthony Shay's *Choreophobia* in *Habibi*.

10 In my discussion on Cypriot nationalism, I rely on Anderson's theory on nations. What is also useful and necessary to acknowledge, though, is that queer theorists have established associations between Anderson's work on nation and queer identity. B.J. Wray employs these associations in "Choreographing Queer": "Anderson's musings on the foundational role of the imagination in the constitution of

all nations provides an obvious theoretical framework for queer speculations on community and citizenship" (30).

11 In *Ours Once More*, Herzfeld argues that Greek folklore was reformulated in studies organized around the theme of cultural continuity to connect modern Greeks with the Western ideological concept of "Hellas." Closer to my concern with movement and performance of gender, Greek folklore would undoubtedly prove fascinating to explore using recent insights from postcolonial theory and gender studies.

12 For more information on the twentieth century history of the *amanes*, the ambivalent treatment of its oriental associations in Greek culture, the *amanes* history in the diasporic communities of Greeks, Arabs, Armenians, and Turks in the United States see Gail Holst-Warhaft's article "Amanes: The Legacy of the Oriental Mother" at <www.muspe.unibo.it> (search for *amanes* from main page). The web site also provides sample *amane* songs.

13 In her article "Amanes: The Legacy of the Oriental Mother," Holst-Warhaft explains that "each makam is not a scale but a group of melodic passages in one or more tone levels," and that "the particular makam will dictate the melodic contour of each amanes" <www.muspe.unibo.it>.

14 The Petrides attempt the same with the karçilama, another dance that is popular in a variety of forms in Greece, Cyprus, and Turkey. They believe it stems from "an ancient Pyrrhic dance, the vestiges of which were preserved by the Byzantines" (27).

15 There exist several good examples of such songs, especially a selection included in *Greek-Oriental Rebetica: Songs and Dances in the Asia Minor Style, 1911–1937*, an important compilation.

16 Writing about Manos Hadjidakis, Holst-Warhaft contends that "the presentation of rebetika to a sophisticated Athenian audience by a man respected as a 'serious' composer marked the beginning of the cultivation of rebetika by a significant group of Greek artists and intellectuals, some of whom, like the painter Tsarouhis, undoubtedly shared Hadjidakis' attraction to the exclusively male environment of the songs" ("Rebetika" 123). Both Tsarouhis and Hadjidakis, however, did not remain spectators but proceeded to produce work (paintings and music respectively) inspired by rebetika.

17 For illustrations and a discussion of Tsarouhis's paintings on the subject of male dancing bodies, see Aphrodite Kouria's article "Thoughts on Some Dance Themes in Modern Greek Painting" 211-15.

18 There have been attempts to claim the zeibekiko as a wholly Greek dance and separate it from its Eastern roots. Katia Savrami, in her article "Two Diverse Versions of the Dance Zeibekiko," makes the claim that the origin of the word "zeibekiko" is Greek rather than Turkish. In the case of the tsifteteli, similar attempts have been few (I mention Petrides and Buccheld in this chapter). A study such as Lawler's *The Dance of the Ancient Greek Theatre*, where she describes dances such as the "cordax" (69-86), the "igdis," the "apokinos," and the "hygros" (72-74), has not provided incentive in the Greek world of dance for a quest for origins of the tsifteteli. The dances that Lawler describes, and which I mention here, feature moves that resemble, quite strikingly, contemporary renditions of belly dance.

19 Since writing this chapter, I have had an interesting and useful exchange with Gail Holst-Warhaft on the issue of parody. I relay part of this exchange since it clarifies

Warhaft's comment with some background information and also contributes some important observations about rebetiko culture in the latter half of the twentieth century. In an e-mail, Warhaft informed me that her remarks concerned scenes she witnessed in various sites in Athens in the 1960s and '70s. The male tsifteteli performance she describes with "men holding their genitals" and gyrating in "a lewd parody of female dancing" was indeed part of her experience. She spoke of a tiny club near Monastiraki, in Athens, where a group of young men used to get together to listen to rebetika on the juke-box and dance. When they had enough money they would go to hear Soteria Bellou (a very famous and popular rebetika singer), but mostly they met after work at "Zoumeli's." According to Warhaft, the parodic dances they did were usually full of fun, and, as Petropoulos describes, they often held their genitals as they danced. As she put it, "I now think that they were not always parodying women, but I find the same phenomenon described in the circles of aficionados of flamenco—men getting together to dance 'as women,' wearing wigs sometimes—and not only gay men. I know men in some areas of Greece, including the Pontian communities of Thrace, dance the tsifteteli with grace and beauty, but in my experience, the dancing of tsifteteli in rebetika circles of Piraeus and Athens, at least in the period when I went to watch it, was parodic. In the fairly exclusively male world of the early bouzouki clubs, tsiftetelia were a rarity, after all. It is later that they formed an important part of the repertoire." And she concludes, with another useful point: "the element of humor and parody was enormously important in rebetika and has, I think, been underestimated" (personal e-mail).

20 This particular documentary was first aired on 21 December 1985. It has been shown a number of times on Greek television since then.

21 I do not wish to demonize the male customers at the cabaret. Their (mostly but not exclusively) lower class status and their predilection for mature women who do not fulfill the supermodel stereotype make them, in fact, somewhat likeable. I feel that the film invites me to see them sympathetically, as people who are at the mercy of circumstance and who can make a woman happy because they are able to respect maturity, experience, and a full female figure. Nevertheless, that Lilia achieves a new awakening when she discovers she can still be sexually attractive to men is not entirely unproblematic. Why should it always be the desiring male heterosexual gaze that affirms a woman's sexuality? In fact, the confirmation and support she receives through her homosocial bonding with the female cabaret dancers, especially Folla, is a lot more engaging but unfortunately underexplored. Moreover, the male hairdresser who is also the singer at the wedding ceremony that I discuss here, has extraordinary potential for disrupting and dismantling the heterosexual dynamic in this film where heterosexual, patriarchal orthodoxy is Lilia's system of oppression. However, his character is not applied to that purpose so the film (indirectly perhaps) validates male heterosexual desire.

22 On the issue of dance in the film and its commercial exploitation for the Greek tourist industry, see Lisbet Torp's article, "Zorba's Dance: The Story of a Dance Illusion – And Its Touristic Value," 207-10.

23 There was also an intransigent quality to Λαϊκή μουσική as contrasted with the demotic or folkloric songs (the Δημοτικά τραγούδια that I refer to in chapter 1). Urban songs of the people (λαϊκό means "of the people") formed a live and transforming culture expressing urgent issues so they were a difficult form for the

authorities to manipulate. Certainly, these songs were impossible to associate with any grand, national ideals and they could not be stretched back to any classical grandeur, even though rebetika and urban songs musical scales derived not only from Eastern musical roads but Byzantine musical scales. Nationalist ideology wrapped traditional folk songs in an aura of sepia and historicity but this could not become the mode of presentation for urban songs of the people.

24   In fact, the timbre of Kazantzides's voice resonated in the hearts of many Greeks and marked profoundly the Greek psyche and culture. His massive popularity along with the fact that his discography has been enormous makes him arguably the most important Greek singer of modern times. Gail Holst-Warhaft captures Kazantzides's impact in this brief description: "His voice would epitomise the singers of the low-class dives known as *skiladhika*, the haunts of truck-drivers and other nocturnal workers. It was a late-night, heart-on-the sleeve despairing voice, well-suited to the songs of the day that were called 'Turko-gypsy' or 'gypsy' not only because of their use of erotic subject matter but because of their preference for the tsifteteli. Accompanied by a toumbeleki [a small hand drum] and violin, Kazantizides sounds like the generic middle eastern singer found in nightclubs from Tel Aviv to Port Said" ("World Music and the Orientalising of the Rebetika").

25   The most popular rhythms common in both Greek tsifteteli and Egyptian Raqs Sharqi are the *malfoof* and the *maqsoom*. Hossam Ramzy explains and plays these rhythms in the recording *Introduction to Egyptian Dance Rhythms*. Often, not only the specific rhythms but also entire musical phrases are identical in Greek, Arabic, and Turkish songs. Such coincidence should be expected since the musical modes, or *maqams*, are shared between Greeks, Turks, Arabs, and even Iranians. Also necessary to point out is the borrowing that has been taking place between Arabic, Greek, and Turkish musical cultures. For example, Mohammed Abdul Wahab's popular song "Habibi Lasmar" became "Ο Ταυρομάχος μου" ["The Bullfighter"] sung by Yiota Lydia in the late 1950s. More recently, Lefteris Pantazis, a Greek singer of Pontic descent, recorded two songs by Hakim, who is currently one of Egypt's most popular artists. Greeks regard these renditions with the same dubious attention that meets the tsifteteli as a musical genre. This ambivalence is strongly felt in the case of a recent Turkish song by Tarkan, which has been a popular success not only in Turkey but also in Greece. Tarkan has his Greek equivalent in Sakis Rouvas, a singer who has caused some controversy in Greece over his sexual image and his live-in-concert collaboration with Tarkan himself. Although I do not value Rouvas's musical production (mostly overproduced pop songs with no "flavour"), I do appreciate the controversy that his image has stirred. For a discussion of Tarkan's image in Turkey and his ambiguous sexual performance, see Emma Sinclair-Webb "Our Bülent is now a Commando" (65-91). I find it also important to point out that, in more recent times, this interactive relationship between Middle Eastern cultures has been directed, to a certain extent, by the latest transmutations of Orientalism where "Eastern" exotica has become trendy (sometimes this exotica is marked by vague signifiers, such as an Eastern melody emerging syncopated through the beat of a techno dance song). Lefteris Pantazis, and other Greek singers who are in the music business for commercial success, now record Arabic songs motivated more by the wish to be hip and sell records, than to establish musical connections with cultural relations. In

marked contrast to this Orientalist craze is a generation of Greek song writers who approach Eastern musical roads and rhythms with a great deal of expertise as well as sensitivity. Approaching their art with a lyrical disposition, these song writers realize Eastern expressive possibilities in songs that are profoundly intro-spective and often philosophical. Nikos Xydakis (a Greek from Egypt), Tassos Gkrous, and Sokratis Malamas are three representatives of this generation of song-writers. In their compositions, the karçilama and the tsifteteli (rebetika styles in general) are employed for their expressive potential—not merely to entertain or promote a feeling of ephemeral joy. Particularly Xydakis has ren-dered *maqams*, rhythms, and also instruments not only sensitively but with a confidence that revises the *malfoof*, for example, giving it a new hypostasis in the sung culture of Greece. Perhaps Xydakis's upbringing in Cairo and Alexan-dria has played its part in the development of his sensibility and remarkable treat-ment of "Oriental" sounds and traditional instruments of the Eastern Mediterranean. His Alexandrian influences aside, Xydakis has recuperated cer-tain forms of musical expression making it possible for others like Malamas and Gkrous to contribute compositions that expand the concept of what "Greek music" is expected to sound like. The politics as well as the artistry of these com-posers are important in my discussion here.

Notes to Chapter 6

1 In an article entitled "Dance and Jurisprudence in the Islamic Middle East," Anthony Shay challenges the most common Western stereotypes of Islam as cul-ture and religion, and attacks some of the widespread misconceptions about East-ern dance practices.

2 I am thinking specifically of disconcerting but very popular representations: head-less torsos on album covers (an eerie evocation of the decapitated Salomé) and playful women, scantily clad, lying in wanton postures, displaying a disturbing availability. "Voice of Stars" is a music label that has brought out some remark-able collections of Oriental dance music but its album covers have depicted female performers in poses and costumes that are, if not quite pornographic, clearly fetishistic and certainly compromising.

3 For further elaboration on this point, see Barbara Sellers Young's article "Raks El Sharki: Transculturation of a Folk Form."

4 In a television documentary, which I cannot unfortunately cite by title and date of broadcast, I watched a woman recounting her past as an overweight, bulimic person who found solace and meaning for her physical existence in belly dance. It was an emotionally charged account and hers is not the only one. Hundreds of women benefit from this particular dance and are able to make a fresh start with a revived interest in their mental and physical health. This dance is not vindictive on the body in the sense that what it is capable of expressing does not require any particular physique or an early beginning in childhood or adoles-cence. It can, therefore, offer a great deal to anyone who is willing to devote time and energy. Raja Amari's film *Satin Rouge* gives a universal twist to the lib-erating and rejuvenating potential of belly dance. The film's central theme is Lilia's journey of self discovery, a widowed and lonely mother from Tunis. She is able to reinvent her body and her sexuality, and escape the void in her life after

becoming a belly dance performer on the stage of a low-class cabaret in her part of the city. Although it handles its theme with respect and delicacy, the film at times exaggerates the euphoria that overtakes male viewers and female performers at the cabaret where Lilia ends up performing.

5 Marianna Torgovnick's *Gone Primitive* is one of the most useful and comprehensive psychoanalytic studies on the primitive and its political and artistic implications.

6 Moreover, Raftis's exclamation and prompting seem unconsious of the fact that his comments on the misunderstandings about Greek dance (I cite and comment on these in chapter 5, note 2) remain largely—and sadly—unaddressed seventeen years after the publication of *The World of Greek Dance*, where he alludes to Dora Stratou and her "naïve treatment [that] covers with a dose of facile patriotism the nonexistence of serious study on modern Greek dance" (*The World of Greek Dance* 22).

7 In personal communication, Yasmina Ramzy helped clarify this point with some interesting insights on American belly dance interpretations. She agrees that Jillina has great talent and enormous skill and finds Jillina's technique to be Arabic. The contrast that Ramzy generally discerns between North American interpretations of belly dance and those of indigenous dancers in the Middle East is in the *presentation* of the dance. North American choreographies often project outwards with an emphasis on being intelligible for the general public, hence the "cheerleader quality" of some American belly dance performances. In the Middle East, however, the presentation is internal, with the dancer focused within and communicating a range of personal emotions to an audience that expects a complex emotional transformation from her performance. If I understand Ramzy's point, the terms "exoteric" and "esoteric" would be appropriate to describe the contrast, especially because of their respective associations with spectacle and ritual that I discuss in chapter 3. In this contrast lies the reason why North American choreographies are often varied and very elaborate whereas an Egyptian or Lebanese dancer, for example, will repeat the same move through much of the routine and only occasionally vary it with her "signature" moves. Her audience is already initiated, with strong reference points for her performance while the expectation is not merely to be entertained. I realize that such an attempt to "fix" the characters of belly dance presentations in East and West may engender various political complications. Nonetheless, I find the distinction useful when used in a heuristic manner, i.e., once we articulate it then we can proceed to challenge it and/or explore deeper understandings of the cultural implications of an Eastern dance performed on the Western stage. Finally on this point, Ali Jihad Racy has produced a brilliant study on *tarab*, the act of spiritual intoxication of both audience members and performers during a performance. Although in his book *Making Music in the Arab World: The Culture and Artistry of Tarab*, Racy does not focus on the experience of tarab during a dance performance, his discussion would be quite useful in understanding the expectations and the dynamic of performance in the Middle East.

8 I had the opportunity to watch the "Bellydance Superstars and Desert Roses" show in Vancouver on 13 April 2004. Miles Copeland was there to speak and introduce the show. His introduction was distasteful, uninspiring, and unreflective of some of the dancers' level of skill, talent, and emotional investment in the art.

However, to watch belly dance onstage in a packed theatre felt quite overwhelming. Some of the dancers displayed such skill and artistry that they kept the audience spellbound. It was fascinating that these were American dancers dancing to Arabic singers and Arabic lyrics at a time when American troops are occupying Iraq. Overall, however, the physical distance between performers and audience and the separation imposed by the stage absorbed some of the dance's vital interactive quality. It remains to be seen whether this will help the art form evolve or whether it will be yet another wave of Orientalism, although there is already a voice of concern from the belly dance community that this will be another case of exploitation and appropriation by a Hollywood producer.

9 Unofficial information from a friend in Greece tells me that Eleonora is Bulgarian but this is not confirmed. It has been difficult to track down information on this dancer.

10 For a detailed look at the history and the etymology of the zar, see Magda Saleh (156-70).

11 Good examples of dancing stillness are the popular statue of Shiva as "The King of Dance (Nataraja)" and "Shiva's Victory Dance." Statue photos are reproduced in Pal Pratapaditya's *Dancing to the Flute* (49 and 53 respectively). The same book includes a photo of the beautifully androgynous Ram Gopal performing at the Channakesava temple in Belur, Karnataka, India (circa 1936). Although a still pose, there is dance flowing through Gopal's body.

12 Rahimieh's project also aims at critiquing Oriental men's complicity with the West's exploitation of Oriental women. Both East and West shared in the oppression: "in the case of Oriental women and their treatment at the hands of Europeans the Oriental societies are, by no means, to be regarded as powerless" (41).

Notes to Epilogue

1 E-mail to the author, 8 November 2003.

2 "Gay Murder in Jigawa" <allafrica.com> 22 April 2002. There is also a link to this news item on a website called "Behind the Mask," a website on gay and lesbian affairs in Africa. (Search under "Africa by country" for Nigeria, "Gay Murder in Jigawa" <www.mask.org.za> 17 October 2004.)

3 One of the interviewees in John Scagliotti's film *Dangerous Living: Coming Out in the Developing World* is Kenny Wellington, a gay man from Namibia and now in London, whose words are reminiscent of Innua Yakubu. Wellington describes the constant threat he felt because of his very movement: "Gay people in the north, in the rural areas got beaten up. We just got frightened. I got frightened of walking around by myself. There's one thing, I can't stop my hips swinging from left to right. If you like it, you like it.... If I respond to an insult, just walking past, I'm just looking for trouble. Walk. Walk away" ("Collected Interviews from the Subjects of *Dangerous Living*" <www.afterstonewall.com> 17 October 2004). The film's focus is to bring to the forefront the often ruthless persecution of people with alternative sexualities. It makes an extremely significant contribution in the dialogue on globalization and sexualities. However, while seriously engaged with its goal, the film, perhaps inadvertently, pushes for the global homogenization of queer sexualities. Because it approaches its subject from the Western position (and, clearly, we are meant to see the West as developed and,

therefore, superior to these still developing places), the film expects us to understand cross-dressing in the Philippines, for example, in terms of cross-dressing in the United States. Another problem is that a huge geographical expanse is termed "developing world" and depicted as harsh, inhuman, and uncivilized when it comes to alternative sexualities. There is no attempt to delineate differences in the approach between the various countries which are, instead, conflated into one barbaric and oppressive system. Of course, the emphasis on "development" in the film's title points to capitalist progress as the standard of comparison, thus making the globalization of sexuality a corollary of Western capitalist society. Finally, since most of the "developing world" interviewees fled from their home to countries such as Britain, the United States, and Canada, the film indirectly champions the West as liberal and progressive, a place where freedoms and human rights are observed and respected, and where asylum is offered generously. Thus, the West does not need to examine its own responsibility in the instigation of homophobia and sexual oppression in the previously colonized nations, or the hate crimes that occur almost daily in the streets, parks, and homes of the "developed world."

4 The lyrics of this song are by Roza Eskenazy and the music by Dimitrios Manisalis. I thank Stelios Lambropoulos for providing me with this information.

5 Mesaoria (literally "in-between mountains") is a large fertile plain that extends from the centre of the island to almost its entire southeastern side. Much of it remains under occupation by Turkish troops.

6 Abdel Halif Hafez, "Gana el Hawa." The lyrics are by Mohammed Hamza and music by Baligh Hamdy.

Works Cited

Ahmad, Aijaz. *In Theory: Classes, Nations, Literatures.* London: Verso, 1992.

Ahmed, Leila. *Women and Gender in Islam: Historical Roots of a Modern Debate.* New Haven: Yale UP, 1992.

Ali, Wijdan. "Modern Painting in the Mashriq." *Colors of Enchantment: Theater, Dance, Music, and the Visual Arts of the Middle East.* Ed. Sherifa Zuhur. Cairo: American U in Cairo P, 2001. 363-85.

Alloula, Malek. *The Colonial Harem.* Trans. Myrna Godzich and Wlad Godzich. Minneapolis: U of Minnesota P, 1986.

And, Metin. *A Pictorial History of Turkish Dancing: From Folk Dancing to Whirling Dervishes—Belly Dancing to Ballet.* Ankara: Dost Yayinlari, 1976.

Anderson, Benedict. *Imagined Communities: Reflections on the Origin and Spread of Nationalism.* Rev. ed. London: Verso 1991.

Anoyiannakis, Phoivos. Ελληνικά Λαικά Μουσικά Οργανα [*Greek Folk Musical Instruments*]. Athens: Melissa, 1976.

Behdad, Ali. *Belated Travelers: Orientalism in the Age of Colonial Dissolution.* Durham: Duke UP, 1994.

Berger, Morroe. "The Arab Danse du Ventre." *Dance Perspectives* 10 (1961): 1-49.

Bernal, Martin. *Black Athena: The Afroasiatic Roots of Classical Civilization.* Vol. 1: *The Fabrication of Ancient Greece 1785-1985.* New Brunswick: Rutgers UP, 1987.

Bhabha, Homi. *The Location of Culture.* London: Routledge, 1994.

Boone, Joseph. "Vacation Cruises; or, The Homoerotics of Orientalism." *Postcolonial, Queer: Theoretical Intersections.* Ed. John C. Hawley. New York: State U of New York P, 2001. 43-78.

Buchheld, Ulf. "Περί της τού Τσιφτετελιού Προελεύσεως" ["Concerning the Origins of the Tsifteteli"]. *Dance and Ancient Greece.* Ed. Alkis Raftis and Anna Lazou. Athens: Way of Life, 1991. 30-59.

Buck, Elizabeth. "Rakkasah—An American Middle Eastern Dance Festival: Exoticism and Orientalism in the Twentieth Century." *UCLA Journal of Dance Ethnology* 15 (1991): 26-32.

221

Buonaventura, Wendy. *The Serpent of the Nile: Women and Dance in the Arab World*. London: Saqi, 1989.

Burt, Ramsay. *The Male Dancer: Bodies, Spectacles, Sexualities*. London: Routledge, 1995.

Burton, Richard F. "Terminal Essay." *A Plain and Literal Translation of the Arabian Nights' Entertainments, Now Entituled The Book of the Thousand Nights and a Night, with Introduction Explanatory Notes on the Manners and Customs of Moslem Men and a Terminal Essay upon the History of the Nights*. Vol. 10. London: Burton Club, 1886. 63-302.

———, et al. "Supplement to Vol. 1." *The Arabian Nights Entertainments*. Vol 1. New York: Macy, 1955. 1-136.

Carlton, Donna. *Looking for Little Egypt*. Bloomington: IDD, 1994.

Cherniavsky, Felix. *The Salomé Dancer: The Life and Times of Maud Allan*. Toronto: McClelland and Stewart, 1991.

Chow, Rey. "Where Have All the Natives Gone?" *Contemporary Postcolonial Theory: A Reader*. Ed. Padmini Mongia. London: Arnold, 1996. 122-46.

Clerides, Nearhos. "Κυπριακοί Χοροί : Λεβεντιά και Σεμνότης" ["The Dances of Cyprus: Valour and Decency"]. *Eleftheria* 13 May 1961: 4.

Coco, Carla. *Secrets of the Harem*. London: Philip Wilson, 1997.

Colette. *Places*. Trans. David Le Vay. London: Peter Owen, 1970.

Covel, John. "Extracts from the Diaries of Dr. John Covel, 1670-1679." *Early Voyages and Travels in the Levant*. Ed. Theodore Bent. New York: Burt Franklin. 99-287.

Crompton, Louis. *Byron and Greek Love: Homophobia in Nineteenth-Century England*. London: Faber and Faber, 1985.

Curtis, George William. *Nile Notes of a Howadji*. New York: Dix, Edwards, 1857.

Dahlin, Dondi Simone. "On Being a Superstar—Dondi's Tour Diary." <www.bellydancesuperstars.com>

Danielson, Virginia. *The Voice of Egypt: Umm Kulthum, Arabic Song, and Egyptian Society in the Twentieth Century*. Cairo: American U in Cairo P, 1997.

Daoud, Hassan. "Those Two Heavy Wings of Manhood: On Moustaches." *Imagined Masculinities: Male Identity and Culture in the Middle East*. Ed. Mai Ghoussoub and Emma Sinclair-Webb. London: Saqi, 2000. 273-80.

Deagon, Andrea. "Dance, Body, Universe." *Habibi* 15.2 (Spring 1996): 16-17, 27.

———. "The Dance of the Seven Veils." Forthcoming in *Belly Dance: Representation, Orientalism, and Harem Fantasy*. Ed. Anthony Shay and Barbara Sellers Young. Middletown, CT: Wesleyan UP.

———. "Feminism and Belly Dance." *Habibi* 17.4 (Fall 1999): 8-13.

———. "Framing the Ancient History of Oriental Dance." *Habibi* 19.3 (July 2003): 32-41.

———. "The Image of the Eastern Dancer: Flaubert's Salomé." *Habibi* 19.1 (January 2002): 10-18.

———. "Inanna's Descent: An Archetype of Feminine Self-Discovery and Transformation." *Habibi* 14.3 (Summer 1995): 16-19.

————. "Mythology and Symbolism in Middle Eastern Dance." *Habibi* 16.3 (Summer 1997): 7-11.

De Lauretis, Teresa. "Film and the Visible." *How Do I Look? Queer Film and Video.* Ed. Bad Object Choices. Seattle: Bay, 1991. 223-76.

Denon, Vivant. *Travels in Upper and Lower Egypt, in Company with Several Divisions of the French Army, During the Campaigns of General Bonaparte in that Country.* Trans. Arthur Aikin. Vol. 1. 1803. London: Arno, 1973.

Desmond, Jane. "Dancing out the Difference: Cultural Imperialism and Ruth St. Denis's 'Radha' of 1906." *Signs: Journal of Women in Culture and Society* 17.1 (Autumn 1991): 28-49.

————. "Embodying Difference: Issues of Dance in Dance and Cultural Studies." *Meaning in Motion: New Cultural Studies of Dance.* Ed. Jane Desmond. Durham: Duke UP, 1997. 29-54.

————. "Introduction. Making the Invisible Visible: Staging Sexualities Through Dance." *Dancing desires: Choreographing Sexualities On and Off the Stage.* Ed. Jane Desmond. Wisconsin: U of Wisconsin P, 2001. 3-32.

————, ed. *Meaning in Motion: New Cultural Studies of Dance.* Durham: Duke UP, 1997.

Diogenis. "Η Σάτιρα της Ημέρας: Η Μαρίζα" ["The Satire of the Day: Mariza"]. *Fileleftheros* 7 April 1976: 1.

Dolan, Jill. "In Defense of the Discourse: Materialist Feminism, Postmodernism, Poststructuralism ... and Theory." *Presence and Desire: Essays on Gender, Sexuality and Performance.* Ann Arbor: U of Michigan P, 1993. 85-97.

Drousiotis, Makarios. Η Σκοτεινή Όψη *[EOKA: The Dark Side].* Athens: Stahi, 1998.

Duncan, James, and Derek Gregory, eds. *Writes of Passage: Reading Travel Writing.* London: Routledge, 1999.

Durrell, Lawrence. *Bitter Lemons of Cyprus.* London: Faber and Faber, 1959.

Edwards, Amelia. *A Thousand Miles Up the Nile.* 1899. London: Parkway, 1993.

Ellis, Sylvia C. *The Plays of W.B. Yeats: Yeats and the Dancer.* New York: St. Martin's, 1995.

El-Safy, Shareen. "Raqs Sharqi: Cairo's Disappearing Act." *Habibi* 17.4 (December 1999): 32-38.

Eskenazy, Roza. Αυτά Που Θυμάμαι *[What I Remember].* Ed. Kostas Hatzidoulis. Athens: Kaktos, 1982.

Fahmy, Farida (Melda). "The Creative Development of Mahmoud Reda, a Contemporary Egyptian Choreographer." MA Thesis. U of California at Los Angeles, 1987.

Fanon, Frantz. *Black Skin, White Masks.* Trans. Charles Lam Markmann. New York: Grove, 1967.

Fink, Jennifer Natalya. "Conclusion. Pushing through the Surface: Notes on Hybridity and Writing." *Performing Hybridity.* Ed. May Joseph and Jennifer Natalya Fink. Minneapolis: U of Minnesota P, 1999. 247-52.

Finney, Gail. "The (Wo)Man in the Moon: Wilde's Salomé." *Women in Modern Drama; Freud, Feminism and European Theater at the Turn of the Century.* Ithaca: Cornell UP, 1989.

Flaubert, Gustave. *The Letters of Gustave Flaubert: 1830-1857.* Trans. Francis Steegmuller. Cambridge: Belknap, 1980.

———. "Herodias." *Three Tales.* Trans. Robert Baldick. Harmondsworth: Penguin, 1961. 89-124.

Fone, Byrne. *Homophobia: A History.* New York: Picador, 2000.

Forster, E.M. *A Room with a View.* Harmondsworth: Penguin, 1978.

Foster, Susan Leigh, et al. Introduction. *Corporealities: Dancing Knowledge, Culture and Power.* London: Routledge, 1996. xi-xvii.

———. "Choreographies of Gender." *Signs: Journal of Women in Culture and Society* 24.1 (1998): 1-33.

———. "Choreographing History." *Choreographing History.* Bloomington: Indiana UP, 1995.

Franken, Marjorie. "Farida Fahmy and the Dancer's Image in Egyptian Film." *Images of Enchantment: Visual and Performing Arts of the Middle East.* Ed. Sherifa Zuhur. Cairo: American U in Cairo P, 1998. 265-81.

Fraser, Kathleen Wittick. "The Aesthetics of Belly Dance: Egyptian-Canadians Discuss the Baladi." MFA Thesis. York U, Toronto, ON, 1991.

———. "Public and Private Entertainment at a Royal Egyptian Wedding: 1845." *Habibi* 19.1 (January 2002): 36-38.

Freud, Sigmund. "Mourning and Melancholia." *On Metapsychology: The Theory of Psychoanalysis.* Trans. James Strachey. Ed. Angela Richards. Middlesex: Penguin, 1985. 251-68.

"A Gay Murder in Jigawa." <allafrica.com> 22 April 2002.

Garber, Marjorie. *Vested Interests: Cross-Dressing and Cultural Anxiety.* New York: Harper Perennial, 1992.

Garelick, Rhonda K. *Rising Star: Dandyism, Gender, and Performance in the Fin de Siècle.* Princeton: Princeton UP, 1998.

Georgiades, Nearhos. Το Φαινόμενο Τσιτσάνης [*The Tsitsanis Phenomenon*]. Athens: Sighroni Epohi, 2001.

Ghoussoub, Mai, and Emma Sinclair-Webb, eds. *Imagined Masculinities: Male Identity and Culture in the Middle East.* London: Saqi, 2000.

Gide, André. *Amyntas: North African Journals.* Trans. Richard Howard. New York: Echo, 1988.

Gold, Kerry. "Belly dance goes mass market: Impresario turns a folk dance into a successful onstage extravaganza." *Vancouver Sun* 8 April 2004. C14-5.

Gourgouris, Stathis. *Dream Nation: Enlightenment, Colonization, and the Institution of Modern Greece.* Stanford: Stanford UP, 1996.

Gregory, Derek. "Scripting Egypt: Orientalism and the Cultures of Travel." *Writes of Passage: Reading Travel Writing.* Ed. James Duncan and Derek Gregory. London: Routledge, 1998. 114-50.

Grewal, Inderpal. *Home and Harem: Nation, Gender, Empire, and Cultures of Travel.* Durham: Duke UP, 1996.

Hamilton, Lady Augusta. *Marriage, Rites, Customs and Ceremonies of All Nations of the Universe.* London: Chapple and Son, 1822.

Hanna, Judith Lynne. *Dance, Sex, and Gender: Signs of Identity, Dominance, Defiance, and Desire.* Chicago: U of Chicago P, 1988.

Hawley, John C., ed. *Postcolonial, Queer: Theoretical Intersections.* New York: State U of New York P, 2001.

Hawthorne, Melanie. "'Comment Peut-on Être Homosexuel?' Multinational (In)Corporation and the Frenchness of *Salomé.*" *Perennial Decay: On the Aesthetics and Politics of Decadence.* Ed. Liz Constable, Dennis Denisoff, and Matthew Potolsky. Philadelphia: U of Philadelphia P, 1999. 159-82.

Herzfeld, Michael. "Hellenism and Occidentalism: The Permutations of Performance in Greek Bourgeois Identity." *Occidentalism: Images of the West.* Ed. James G. Carrier. Oxford: Clarendon, 1995. 218-33.

———. *Ours Once More: Folklore, Ideology, and the Making of Modern Greece.* Austin: U of Texas P, 1982.

Hoare, Philip. *Wilde's Last Stand: Decadence, Conspiracy and the First World War.* London: Duckworth, 1997.

Holst, Gail. *Road to Rembetika: Music of a Greek Sub-culture—Songs of Love, Sorrow and Hashish.* Evia: Denise Harvey, 1994.

Holst-Warhaft, Gail. "Amanes: The Legacy of the Oriental Mother" <www .muspe.unibo.it> 17 October 2004.

———. "Rebetika: The Double-Descended Deep Songs of Greece." *Passion of Music and Dance: Body, Gender, and Sexuality.* Ed. William Washabaugh. Oxford: Berg, 1998. 111-26.

———. "Song, Self-Identity, and the Neohellenic." *Journal of Modern Greek Studies* 15.2 (1997): 232-38.

———. "World Music and the Orientalising of the Rebetika." Hydra Rebetiko Conference, Hydra, Greece, 2001. (Archive of Rebetika-related material <www.geocities.com/hydragathering> 17 October 2004.)

hooks, bell. *Black Looks: Race and Representation.* Toronto: Between the Lines, 1992.

Janssen, Thijs. "Transvestites and Transsexuals in Turkey." *Sexuality and Eroticism among Males in Moslem Societies.* Ed. Arno Schmitt and Jehoeda Sofer. New York: Haworth, 1992.

Johnson, Frank Edward. "Here and There in Northern Africa." *National Geographic* 25.1 (1914): 1-132.

Jonas, Gerald. *Dancing: The Pleasure, Power, and Art of Movement.* NY: Harry N. Abrams, 1992.

Joseph, May, and Jennifer Natalya Fink, eds. *Performing Hybridity.* Minneapolis: U of Minnesota P, 1999.

Kabbani, Rana. *Europe's Myths of Orient: Devise and Rule.* London: Macmillan, 1986.

Kamboureli, Smaro. *Scandalous Bodies: Diasporic Literature in English Canada.* Don Mills: Oxford UP, 2000.

Kealiinohomoku, Joann. "An Anthropologist Looks at Ballet as a Form of Ethnic Dance." *What Is Dance? Readings in Theory and Criticism.* Ed. Roger Copeland and Marshall Cohen. Oxford: Oxford UP, 1983. 533-49.

Koestenbaum, Wayne. *The Queen's Throat: Opera, Homosexuality, and the Mystery of Desire.* New York: Vintage, 1993.

Koritz, Amy. "Dancing the Orient for England: Maud Allan's *The Vision of Salomé.*" *Meaning in Motion: New Cultural Studies of Dance.* Ed. Jane Desmond. Durham: Duke UP, 1997. 133-52.

———. "Oscar Wilde's *Salomé*: Rewriting the Fatal Woman." *Gendering Bodies/Performing Art: Dance and Literature in Early Twentieth-Century British Culture.* Ann Arbor: U of Michigan P, 1995. 75-85.

Kouria, Afrodite. "Thoughts on Some Dance Themes in Modern Greek Painting." Εθνογραφικά: Ο Χορός στην Ελλάδα *[The Dance in Greece].* Vol. 8. Ed. Rena Loutzaki. Nafplio: Peloponnesian Folklore Foundation, 1992. 211-14.

Lane, Edward. W. *Manners and Customs of the Modern Egyptians.* London: Everyman, 1966.

Lawler, Lillian B. *The Dance of the Ancient Greek Theatre.* Iowa: U of Iowa P, 1964.

———. "Terpsichore: The Story of Dance in Ancient Greece." *Dance Perspectives* (Winter 1962): 2-57.

Leland, Charles G. *The Egyptian Sketchbook.* London: Strahan, Trubner, 1873.

Lentakis, Andreas. Ιερά Πορνεία *[Sacred Prostitution].* Athens: Dorikos, 1990.

Lewis, Reina. *Gendering Orientalism: Race, Femininity and Representation.* London: Routledge, 1996.

Lexová, Irena. *Ancient Egyptian Dances.* Trans. K. Haltmar. 1935. Mineola, NY: Dover, 2000.

Loomba, Ania. *Colonialism/Postcolonialism.* London: Routledge, 1998.

Lorius, Cassandra. "'Oh Boy, You Salt of the Earth': Outwitting Patriarchy in *Raqs Baladi.*" *Popular Music* 15.3 (1996): 285-98.

Loutzaki, Rena. Ed. Εθνογραφικά: Ο Χορός στην Ελλάδα *[The Dance in Greece].* Vol. 8. Nafplio: Peloponnesian Folklore Foundation, 1992.

Lowe, Lisa. *Critical Terrains: French and British Orientalisms.* Ithaca: Cornell UP, 1991.

Marchand, Leslie A. Ed. *"In My Hot Youth": Byron's Letters and Journals.* Vol. 1: 1798-1810. London: Murray, 1973.

McClintock, Anne. *Imperial Leather: Race, Gender and Sexuality in the Colonial Contest.* London: Routledge, 1995.

Mernissi, Fatima. *Beyond the Veil: Male-Female Dynamics in Modern Muslim Society.* Cambridge: Schenkman, 1975.

Mitchell, Timothy. *Colonising Egypt.* Berkeley: U of California P, 1988.

Montague, Lady Mary Wortley. *Letters from the Levant during the Embassy to Constantinople 1716-18. 1838.* New York: Arno, 1971.

Monty, Paul Eugene. "Serena, Ruth St. Denis, and the Evolution of Belly Dance (1876-1976)." PhD dissertation. New York U, 1986.

Moore-Gilbert, Bart. *Postcolonial Theory; Contexts, Practices, Politics.* London: Verso, 1997.

Murray, Stephen, and Will Roscoe, eds. *Islamic Homosexualities: Culture, History, and Literature.* New York: New York UP, 1997.

Murray, Stephen. "The Will Not to Know." *Islamic Homosexualities: Culture, History, and Literature.* Eds. Stephen Murray and Will Roscoe. New York: New York UP, 1997. 14-54.

Nerval, Gerard de. *The Women of Cairo: Scenes of Life in the Orient.* London: Routledge, 1929.

Nieuwkerk, Karin van. *"A Trade Like Any Other:" Dancers and Courtesans in Egypt.* Austin: U of Texas P, 1995.

Ohnefalsch-Richter, Magda. *Griechische Sitten und Gebräuche auf Cypern* [*Greek Customs and Traditions of Cyprus*]. Trans. Anna Marangou. Nicosia: Cyprus Popular Bank Cultural Centre, 1994.

Orga, Irfan. *The Caravan Moves On: Three Weeks among Turkish Nomads.* London: Eland, 2002.

Özdemir, Kemal. *Oriental Belly Dance.* Istanbul: Dönence Basim ve Yayin Hizmetleri, 2000.

Peckham, Shannan Robert. "The Exoticism of the Familiar and the Familiarity of the Exotic: Fin-de-Siècle Travellers to Greece." *Writes of Passage: Reading Travel Writing.* Ed. James Duncan and Derek Gregory. London: Routledge, 1999. 164-84.

Petrides, Theodore, and Elfleida Petrides. *Folk Dances of the Greeks.* New York: Exposition, 1961.

Petropoulos Elias. Ρεμπετικα Τραγουδια [*Rebetika Songs*]. Athens: Kedros, 1991.

Phillips, Richard. "Writing Travel and Mapping Sexuality: Richard Burton's Sotadic Zone." *Writes of Passage: Reading Travel Writing.* Ed. James Duncan and Derek Gregory. London: Routledge, 1999. 70-91.

Pizanias, Caterina. "(Re)thinking the Ethnic Body: Performing 'Greekness' in Canada." *Journal of the Hellenic Diaspora* 22.1 (1996): 7-60.

Pratapaditya, Pal, ed. *Dancing to the Flute: Music and Dance in Indian Art.* Sydney: Art Gallery of New South Wales, 1997.

Pratt, Mary Louise. *Imperial Eyes: Travel Writing and Transculturation.* London: Routledge, 1992.

Praz, Mario. *The Romantic Agony.* Trans. Angus Davidson. New York: Meridian, 1960.

Racy, Ali Jihad. *Making Music in the Arab World: The Culture and Artistry of Tarab.* Cambridge: Cambridge UP, 2003.

Rahimieh, Nasrin. *Oriental Responses to the West: Comparative Essays in Select Writers from the Muslim World.* Leiden: E.J. Brill, 1990.

Raftis, Alkis. Ο Κόσμος του Ελληνικού Χορού [The World of Hellenic Dance]. Athens: Polytypos, 1985.

———. Χορός 1900: Οι Ελληνικές ταχυδρομικές κάρτες τών αρχών του αιώνα με θέμα το Χορό [Dance 1900: Turn-of-the-Century Postcards Portraying Dance]. Athens: Tropos Zois, 1999.

Ross, Robert. "A Note on 'Salomé.'" Salomé: A Tragedy in One Act. By Oscar Wilde. New York: Williams, Belasco, and Meyers, 1930. 15-21.

Sachs, Susan. "He's No Salomé, But It's Straight from the Heart." New York Times. 4 May 2000. 28 December 2001. <www.nytimes.com> 28 December 2001.

Said, Edward. Culture and Imperialism. New York: Vintage, 1994.

———. "Farewell to Tahia." Colors of Enchantment: Theater, Dance, Music, and the Visual Arts of the Middle East. Ed. Sherifa Zuhur. Cairo: American U in Cairo P, 2001. 228-32.

———. "Homage to a Belly-Dancer: On Tahia Carioca." Reflections on Exile and Other Essays. Cambridge: Harvard UP, 2000. 346-55.

———. Orientalism. New York: Vintage, 1979.

———. Reflections on Exile and Other Essays. Cambridge: Harvard UP, 2000.

Saleh, Magda Ahmed Abdel Ghaffar. "Documentation of the Ethnic Dance Traditions of the Arab Republic of Egypt." PhD dissertation. New York U, 1979.

Salimpur, Suhaila. "I Remember Nadia." Articles, Press, and Statements. <www.suhaila.com> 25 October 2001.

Savigliano, Marta. Tango and the Political Economy of Passion. Boulder: Westview, 1995.

Savrami, Katia. "Two Diverse Versions of the Dance Zeibekiko." Dance Studies 16 (1992): 57-103.

Scagliotti, John. "Dangerous Living: Primary Interviews." <www.afterstonewall.com> 17 October 2004.

Schuyler, Eugene. Turkistan: Notes of a Journey in Russian Turkistan, Kokand, Bukhara and Kuldja. Ed. Geoffrey Wheeler. New York: Frederick A. Praeger, 1966.

Sedgwick, Eve Kosofsky. Between Men: English Literature and Male Homosocial Desire. New York: Columbia UP, 1985.

———. Epistemology of the Closet. Berkeley: U of California P, 1990.

———. Tendencies. Durham: Duke UP, 1993.

Sellers-Young, Barbara. "Raks El Sharki: Transculturation of a Folk Form." Journal of Popular Culture 26.2 (Fall 1992): 141-52.

Shand, Angela. "The Tsifte-teli Sermon: Identity, Theology, and Gender in Rebetika." Passion of Music and Dance: Body, Gender and Sexuality. Ed. William Washabaugh. Oxford: Berg, 1998. 127-32.

Shay, Anthony. Choreographic Politics: State Folk Dance Ensembles, Representation, and Power. Middletown, CT: Wesleyan UP, 2002.

———. *Choreophobia: Solo Improvised Dance in the Iranian World.* Costa Mesa: Mazda, 1999.

———. "Dance and Jurisprudence in the Islamic Middle East." *Habibi* 19.2 (September 2002): 26-39.

———. "The Male Dancer." Forthcoming in *Belly Dance: Representation, Orientalism, and Harem Fantasy.* Ed. Anthony Shay and Barbara Sellers Young. Middletown, CT: Wesleyan UP.

———. "Parallel Traditions: State Folk Dance Ensembles and Folk Dance in 'The Field'." *Dance Research Journal* 31.1 (Spring 1999): 29-56.

Shohat, Ella. "Notes on the 'Post-Colonial.'" *The Pre-occupation of Postcolonial Studies.* Ed. Fawzia Afzal-Khan and Kalpana Seshadri-Crooks. Durham: Duke UP, 2000. 126-39.

Showalter, Elaine. *Sexual Anarchy: Gender and Culture at the Fin de Siècle.* New York: Viking, 1990.

Sinclair-Webb, Emma. "'Our Bülent Is Now a Commando': Military Service and Manhood in Turkey." *Imagined Masculinities: Male Identity and Culture in the Middle East.* Ed. Mai Ghoussoub and Emma Sinclair-Webb. London: Saqi, 2000. 65-92.

Sladen, Douglas. *Egypt and the English: Showing British public opinion in Egypt upon the Egyptian question; with chapters on the success of the Sudan and the delights of travel in Egypt and the Sudan.* London: Hurst and Blackett, 1908.

Sonnini, Sigisbert Charles. *Travels in Upper and Lower Egypt.* 1800. Farnborough: Gregg, 1972.

Spivak, Gayatri Chakravorty. *A Critique of Postcolonial Reason: Toward a History of the Vanishing Present.* Cambridge: Harvard UP, 1999.

———. *The Postcolonial Critic: Interviews, Strategies, Dialogues.* Ed. Sarah Harasym. New York: Routledge, 1990.

Spurlin, William. "Broadening Postcolonial Studies/Decolonizing Queer Studies: Emerging 'Queer' Identities and Cultures in Southern Africa." *Postcolonial, Queer: Theoretical Intersections.* Ed. John C. Hawley. New York: State U of New York P, 2001. 185-206.

Spyrou, Spyros. "Images of 'The Other': 'The Turk' in Greek Cypriot Children's Imaginations." *Race, Ethnicity and Education* 5.3 (2002): 255-72.

———. "Those on the Other Side: Ethnic Identity and Imagination in Greek-Cypriot Children's Lives." *Children and Anthropology: Perspectives for the Twenty-First Century.* Ed. Helen Schwartzman. Westport: Bergin and Garvey, 2001. 167-85.

Stavrou, Stavros. "Review of *Choreophobia.*" *Habibi* 19.1 (2002): 56-57.

Steegmuller, Francis. *Flaubert in Egypt: A Sensibility on Tour.* London: Bodley Head, 1972.

———, ed. *Flaubert and Madame Bovary: A Double Portrait.* New York: Vintage, 1957.

Stewart, Iris, J. *Sacred Woman, Sacred Dance: Awakening Spirituality through Movement and Ritual.* Rochester: Inner Traditions, 2000.

St. John, James Augustus. *Egypt and Nubia: With Illustrations*. London: Chapman and Hall, 1845.

Stokes, Martin, and Ruth Davis. "Introduction." *Popular Music* 15.3 (1996): 255-57.

Stone, Rebecca. "Cinematic Salomés: An Investigation of Dance and Orientalism in Hollywood Films." *UCLA Journal of Dance Ethnology* 15 (1991): 33-42.

Stratou, Dora. *The Greek Dances: Our Living Link with Antiquity*. Trans. Amy Mims-Argyrakis. Athens: Angelos Klissiounis, 1966.

———. Μία Παράδοση, Μία Περιπέτεια: Οι Ελληνικοί Χοροί [*A Tradition, An Adventure: The Greek Dances*]. Athens: G. Phexe, 1964.

Swanson, Linda. "They Said She Could Dance on a Single Tile." Second International Conference on Middle Eastern Dance. Costa Mesa, CA. 27 May 2001.

Thompson, Spurgeon, Stavros Stavrou Karayanni, Myria Vassiliadou. "Cyprus after History." *Interventions: International Journal of Postcolonial Studies* 6.2 (June 2004): 282-99.

Torgovnick, Marianna. *Gone Primitive: Savage Intellects, Modern Lives*. Chicago: U of Chicago P, 1990.

Torp, Lisbet. "'It's All Greek to Me': The Invention of Pan-Hellenic Dances—and Other Stories." *Telling Reality*. Ed. Michael Chesnutt. Copenhagen: NIF 1992. 273-94.

———. "Zorba's Dance: The Story of a Dance Illusion—And Its Touristic Value." Εθνογραφικά: Ο Χορός στην Ελλάδα [*The Dance in Greece*]. Vol. 8. Ed. Rena Loutzaki. Nafplio: Peloponnesian Folklore Foundation, 1992. 207-10.

Trinh, Minh-Ha T. *Framer Framed*. New York: Routledge, 1992.

Tsianikas, Michalis. Ο Φλωμπέρ στήν Ελλάδα [*Flaubert in Greece*]. Athens: Kastaniotis, 1997.

Tsiolkas, Christos. *Loaded*. Milsons Point: Vintage, 1995.

Tucker, Judith E. *Women in Nineteenth-Century Egypt*. Cambridge: Cambridge UP, 1985.

Washabaugh, William, ed. *Passion of Music and Dance: Body, Gender and Sexuality*. Oxford: Berg, 1998.

Weeks, Jeffrey. *Sex, Politics, and Society: The Regulation of Sexuality since 1800*. London: Longman, 1989.

Wilde Oscar. *Salomé: A Tragedy in One Act: Translated from the French of Oscar Wilde, with Sixteen Drawings by Aubrey Beardsley*. New York: Williams, Belasco and Meyers, 1930.

Wood, Leona, and Anthony Shay. "Danse du Ventre: A Fresh Appraisal." *Dance Research Journal* 8:2 (1976): 18-30.

Wray, B.J. "Choreographing Queer: Nationalism, Citizenship, and Lesbian Dance Clubs." *Dancing Bodies, Living Histories: New Writings about Dance and Culture.* Ed. Lisa Doolittle and Anne Flynn. Banff: Banff Centre, 2000. 22-44.

Young, Robert. *Colonial Desire: Hybridity in Theory, Culture and Race.* London: Routledge, 1995.

———. *White Mythologies: Writing History and the West.* London: Routledge, 1990.

Zagona, Helen Grace. *The Legend of Salomé and the Principle of Art for Art's Sake.* Paris: Minard, 1960.

Zuhur, Sherifa, ed. *Colors of Enchantment: Theater, Dance, Music, and the Visual Arts of the Middle East.* Cairo: American U in Cairo P, 2001.

Discography and Film

Ali, Aisha. *Dances of Egypt.* Videocassette. Associated Research in Arab Folklore.

———. *Dances of North Africa—Volume 1: Morocco and Tunisia.* Videocassette. Associated Research in Arab Folklore, 1995.

———. *Music for the Oriental Dance.* LP. Associated Research in Arab Folklore Records, 1977.

———. *Music of the Ghawazee.* LP. Associated Research in Arab Folklore Records, 1973.

Amari, Raja, Dir. *Satin Rouge.* DVD. Zeitgeist Films, 2002.

Buonaventura, Wendy. *Arabic Dance in Performance: Revelations (The Testament of Salomé) and Dancing Girls.* Videocassette. Cinnabar, 1998.

Dancing. Dir. David Wolff. PBS. Thirteen/WNET, New York. 1993.

Egypt: Music of the Nile from the Desert to the Sea. Various Artists. Compact Disc. Virgin France, 1997.

Greek-Oriental Rebetica: Songs and Dances in the Asia Minor Style, 1911-1937. Compact Disc. New York: Arhoolie, 1991.

Hafez, Abdel Halim. "Gana Alhawa." *An Evening with Abdel Halim Hafez.* Compact Disc. 1969. EMI Music Arabia, 1996.

Jalilah. *Journey of the Gipsy Dancer. Jalilah's Raqs Sharki 3.* Compact Disc. Piranha, 1997.

Koch, Mariza. Παναγιά μου, Παναγιά μου [Mother of God]. LP. Athens: Minos Matsas, 1976.

Kokkinos, Ana, Dir. *Head On.* Film. Australian Film Finance Corporation, 2000.

Loizos, Manos. Ο Δρόμος ["The Street"]. Τα Τραγούδια του Δρόμου [Songs of the Street]. LP. Athens: Minos Matsas, 1974.

Μικρασιάτικοι Σκοποί και Τραγούδια [Tunes and Songs from Asia Minor]. Various Artists. Compact Disc. Polygram, 1995.

Oikonomides, Nikos. Πέρασμα στα Κύθηρα [Passage to Kythera]. Compact Disc. Athens: Myrtia, 1996.

Ramzy, Hossam. *Introduction to Egyptian Dance Rhythms*. Compact Disc. ARC Music, 1995.

Scagliotti, John, Dir. *Dangerous Living: Coming Out in the Developing World*. After Stonewall, 2003.

Wahab, Mohammed Abdel. *Belly Dance: The Music of Mohammed Abdel Wahab*. Compact Disc. Digital Press Hellas, Cairophon Series, 1989.

"Yiota Lydia." Οι Παλιοί Μας Φίλοι [*Our Old Friends*]. Dir. Yiorgos Papastefanou. Elliniki Tileorasi. 21 December 1985.

Index

233

238